Viral Economies

Viral Economies

Bird Flu Experiments in Vietnam

NATALIE PORTER

The University of Chicago Press
Chicago and London

The University of Chicago Press, Chicago 60637
The University of Chicago Press, Ltd., London
© 2019 by The University of Chicago
All rights reserved. No part of this book may be used or reproduced in any manner
whatsoever without written permission, except in the case of brief quotations in
critical articles and reviews. For more information, contact the University of Chicago
Press, 1427 E. 60th St., Chicago, IL 60637.
Published 2019
Printed in the United States of America

28 27 26 25 24 23 22 21 20 19   1 2 3 4 5

ISBN-13: 978-0-226-64880-4 (cloth)
ISBN-13: 978-0-226-64894-1 (paper)
ISBN-13: 978-0-226-64913-9 (e-book)
DOI: https://doi.org/10.7208/chicago/9780226649139.001.0001

Library of Congress Cataloging-in-Publication Data

Names: Porter, Natalie (Natalie H.), author.
Title: Viral economies : bird flu experiments in Vietnam / Natalie Porter.
Description: Chicago ; London : The University of Chicago Press, 2019. | Includes
    bibliographical references and index.
Identifiers: LCCN 2019012689 | ISBN 9780226648804 (cloth : alk. paper) |
    ISBN 9780226648941 (pbk. : alk. paper) | ISBN 9780226649139 (e-book)
Subjects: LCSH: Avian influenza—Vietnam. | Poultry—Virus diseases.
Classification: LCC RA644.16 P674 2019 | DDC 614.5/184—dc23
LC record available at https://lccn.loc.gov/2019012689

♾ This paper meets the requirements of ANSI/NISO Z39.48-1992 (Permanence
of Paper).

Contents

Introduction

Daybreak reaches your ears before your eyes on poultry farms in northern Vietnam. It is announced by low sporadic groans, short bursts of exhalation that almost hesitate to disturb the still night air. But then the grunts begin to multiply, in reverberating echoes that lengthen and converge into a single, pulsating drone as darkness gives way to dawn. It takes a naive listener several seconds to link these sounds to the chickens from which they come, and several more to pick up on the pattern of conversation as scores of hens launch weak, disjointed coos that gain in volume and frequency in an escalating struggle to be heard. As the squawk and response grow progressively louder, their cadence quickens, so that individual cries become difficult to distinguish from one another, losing themselves altogether in a frenzied banter so relentless that it denies any attempt at sleep. If nothing else, the cacophony is a call to action, an auditory assault that rouses you from bed and signals the start of a new day.

An entirely different alarm sounded from Vietnamese poultry farms in 2003, one that announced the dawn, not of a new day, but of a new era in global health. In December, at the tail end of sustained global outbreaks of severe acute respiratory syndrome (SARS), the Vietnamese government declared eleven pediatric cases of respiratory illness in the capital city, Hanoi. After ruling out SARS, epidemiologists traced the infections to the same virus that had appeared on commercial poultry farms in South Korea a month before—a novel strain of H5N1 highly pathogenic avian influenza (HPAI). Bird flu.[1] Although H5N2 was not a new virus, its reemergence so quickly after the SARS emergency startled public health officials. Days later, officials announced the appearance of H5N1 again on poultry farms in Vietnam, and by the end of the month they had proclaimed more than four hundred outbreaks in domestic fowl. Outbreak reports rang further and further afield, and in a matter of weeks the virus had broadcast to Japan, Thailand, Cambodia, Laos, Indonesia, and China. Echoing the reports was a growing clamor among international health officials who had never seen H5N1 infect so many countries at the same time. By February, they were sounding off about the possibility of human-to-human virus transmission in Vietnam, a terrifying prospect given the virus's 60 percent mortality rate. By spring, forty-four million birds had been slaughtered across the country.

Like early morning coos and caws, bird flu viruses move quickly through poultry flocks, increasing in volume and range as they communicate across bodily surfaces and secretions. What seems like a mild illness in one bird can erupt as a scourge in others as the rate of infection rises. Whatever its physical effects, bird flu brings unrelenting and comprehensive death. Through contagion and culling, viral communicability pushes fowl and farmers to their tipping points. Still, the real commotion surrounding bird flu stems not from its conveyance among chickens, but from its capacity to cross species. This is what microbiologists call "viral chatter," and when H5N1 came into human range it alerted the world to its pandemic risk and summoned forth a new cadre of global health workers to confront it.

This book tells the story of that awakening. Since 2003, bird flu outbreaks in Vietnam have destroyed hundreds of millions of chickens and ducks, shocked the poultry economy, and killed over one hundred humans. In this corner of Southeast Asia, where many locate the epicenter of pandemic flu infection (Shortridge and Stuart-Harris 1982), bird flu is putting multiple lives and livelihoods at risk. It is also exposing the fact that human health cannot be addressed in isolation from the livestock economies in which bird flu viruses are embedded. Economies matter for two reasons. First, conditions of poultry production and consumption have facilitated H5N1 outbreaks. Second, global health programs have responded to these outbreaks by expanding their purview to include both humans and live*stock*, which are living beings as well as market labor and commodities. In settings where disease passes from poultry to people, global health is transforming into a more-than-human endeavor. Understanding this transformation and its implications requires exploring the economies that shape bird flu on the ground.

In what follows, I document a series of bird flu control programs from their development in policy arenas in Hanoi, through to their implementation and transformation in poultry farming communities in the northern Red River Delta and southern Mekong Delta. I chart the pathways of transnational scientists, NGO workers, state veterinarians, and poultry farmers as they labor to define and address pandemic disease risks. I also document their successes and failures in order to show that when global health interventions surface in domestic livestock economies, they must balance the agendas of state and multinational actors, and they must weigh the interests of public health against those of commercial agriculture, rural tradition, and scientific innovation.

Taken together, this book reveals an arena of global health policy and practice that is increasingly structured by the patterns of global livestock markets. This means that the standardization of life forms and the circum-scription of human-animal relations, which create the conditions for market uniformity and commodity mobility, are now being implemented in bird flu control programs as a means to safeguard human and nonhuman animal health. And yet, because these interventions encounter myriad other ways of living with poultry in Vietnam, I demonstrate that their outcomes are as unpredictable as the flu virus itself. Vietnam thus surfaces in this account as a site of global health experimentation—a place where the agents and sub-jects of disease control are redefining how to live with each other in an age of pandemic risks.

Locating the Global Pandemic

It may seem curious to consider a pandemic threat from the vantage point of a particular site like Vietnam, since what makes viruses like H5N1 so con-cerning is the fact that they transcend national boundaries. Pandemic threats expose uncomfortable truths—that epidemics are not confined to the "de-veloping" world, and that viruses do not discriminate between the Global North and the Global South, rich and poor. In 2003, a business traveler from China was thought to have spread SARS to guests in a Canadian hotel. Ten years later, an American was thought to have infected a Houston nurse with Ebola after visiting relatives in rural Liberia. These events show just how dif-ficult it is to locate, much less to prevent, emerging and reemerging viruses in any particular territory. Over the last three decades, there has been a growing sense among health experts that globally mobile viruses require thoroughly global responses, responses that surpass the capacity of state institutions act-ing alone. In large part because of infections like avian flu, supranational, multinational, and multilateral institutions are playing a larger role in public health practice worldwide (Adams, Novotny, and Leslie 2008).

It is fair to suggest, then, that pandemics call for new kinds of analyses that look beyond discrete territories, states, and populations; and indeed, re-cent studies attempt to upset traditional forms of ethnography written from within particular locales. These studies focus attention on global movements and transmissions—of virus materials and data, of research and prevention strategies, and of discourses and stories told about emerging infections. They take us through advanced technology laboratories in global metropolitan hubs, where scientists sequence, characterize, and "datafy" viruses (Caduff 2012; MacPhail 2014b); to policy strategizing meetings, where experts weigh in on national security risks (Lakoff 2007, 2017); to public health centers, where epidemiologists track outbreaks worldwide (Keck 2015); to metropolitan ports and hospitals, where health workers do the work of pandemic simulation (Samimian-Darash 2009; Wolf and Hall 2018); to media outlets and transnational forums, where pandemic risks are narrated and debated (Briggs and Nichter 2009; Caduff 2014, 2015; Wald 2008). A key contribution of this scholarship has been to show how a new ethos of preparedness animates global health policies and practices (Lakoff 2017). At a time when health experts are relatively certain that a pandemic will emerge, but are profoundly uncertain about where, when, and how, these accounts reveal how geographically disparate people and institutions come together in global networks and assemblages to predict and prepare for the coming plague.

Yet, even as these anticipatory activities surface in global, networked space, I contend that in some sites, and for some species, the pandemic has already arrived. This is certainly true of Vietnam, which has suffered some of the heaviest losses to bird flu. The country tops the worldwide list of reported poultry outbreaks and ranks third worldwide in terms of human fatalities (World Health Organization 2016). To make matters worse, the status of poultry production as a chief industry in Vietnam has meant that avian flu also threatens the country's economic health. In the first year of H5N1 outbreaks alone, Vietnam lost approximately 1 percent of its gross domestic product to the disease and the related poultry-slaughtering measures (McLeod et al. 2006). Millions of small-scale poultry producers have been pushed out of the industry, and those who have stayed are confronting the added financial and familial costs of implementing new health measures on their farms.

In this book, I want to account for the losses that are already occurring as a result of H5N1, and I turn to Vietnam as a place from which to examine how pandemic flu threats have begun shifting the targets, objectives, and practices of global public health. I am interested in documenting how bird flu governance unfolds on the ground, at everyday sites of health planning and intervention, and in light of actual, devastating outbreaks in both human and nonhuman animals.

To carry out this examination, from 2009 to 2013 I conducted ethnographic research on bird flu control measures at three distinct sites in Vietnam. I began the research in Hanoi, the country's capital and home to the key state, multinational, and nongovernmental organizations working in the field of bird flu control. While there I became involved in a global assemblage of avian flu strategists, whom I interviewed, shadowed at work, and observed carrying out interventions in provincial farming communities. At workshops, conferences, and planning meetings, I encountered foreign consultants, expatriates, and Vietnamese citizens working for supranational, multilateral, and multinational health and development organizations, state health and agriculture agencies, and for-profit, nonprofit, and nongovernmental organizations—each with its own set of humanitarian, market, and philanthropic sensibilities.

This research revealed how bird programs and policies surface in contentious relations between professionals. People working in the arena of bird flu management in Vietnam do so from within particular organizations that have their own agendas. Some organizations want to track and contain viruses; some want to empower farmers; others want to commercialize the livestock sector; some want to improve local health institutions; and still others want to strengthen state influence in multinational health programs. In addition to these organizational agendas, individuals working in bird flu management have their own personal accountabilities and career goals. They may want to move up the ranks of government bureaucracy, or gain a foothold in the international development arena, or merely make a little extra income to send their children to school. I observed how these different agendas and aspirations came together in the daily work of bird flu strategizing. I also found that bird flu governance surfaces in a uniquely Vietnamese rubric. In Hanoi's policy-making arena, virus control is brought into line with economic development agendas and state modernization goals, and all of these proceed under the banner of farmer empowerment. As one transnational planner had it, this is the "business model of disease management," in which entrepreneurial individuals adopt commercial livestock standards, and smallholders unable to compete "will eventually disappear."

But can supporting a few entrepreneurial farmers really achieve global virus control? Can selling farmers on a few devices and productive arrangements actually spark a structural transformation in Vietnam's poultry economy? Can health interventions really launch Vietnam into the international trade in commercial meat? And what of the farmers unable to compete? What actually happens to them? The next segment of my research endeavored to answer these questions. I traveled to Bắc Giang, a rural province in the northern Red River Delta known both for chicken farming and bird flu outbreaks. I lived four months with a family of laying hen producers in a village of just over one hundred households, which I refer to in this book as Placid Pond.

The family comprised part of a kin-based network of farmers that dominated egg production in their commune. Trí, the head of the household, was the son of Ông Đức,[2] the first person in the commune to begin raising chickens following postwar rebuilding strategies and farm collectivization failures. Trí's wife, Thủy, had just returned from a five-year stint as an au pair for a middle-class Taiwanese family and was eagerly using her savings to expand their poultry operations.

Trí, Thủy, and their relatives welcomed me into their home, family networks, and daily activities, and abided my requests to engage in daily farming practices. While Trí sold eggs in neighboring markets, Thủy showed me how to feed the hens, collect their eggs, and clean their coops. I held chickens down to the ground during vaccination measures and cordoned them off on days of disinfection. When they were slaughtered, I washed their body parts and prepared them for cooking. In addition to participating in these activities, I had engaging conversations with the ever-curious Trí. Over cases of Hanoi Beer, he lobbied endless questions about chicken farms in the United States and he asked for help translating foreign poultry-keeping guides and veterinary pharmaceutical labels. In turn, he explained Vietnamese poultry market chains and price fluctuations, and he described the familial obligations and reciprocal relations that both facilitated and limited his family's expanding business.

I encountered a different atmosphere during the final stage of my research, when I moved south to Đồng Tháp Province in the Mekong Delta, a region rich in duck farms and bird flu outbreaks. As in Bắc Giang, I had hoped to live with a duck-farming family and participate in daily production activities. But I was immediately assigned to a government minder, Hạnh, a state-employed veterinarian who accompanied me during all of my activities.[3] Realizing that Hạnh's presence would influence any research I conducted with a duck-farming family, I shifted my focus, and turned to Hạnh as a person who could teach me about the work of flu control in settings far removed from central policy-making arenas. Hạnh and I spent many weeks on her motorbike visiting farms and talking to producers, stopping for lunches and coffees to chat about our lives, our families, and our work. She was a consummate professional, the most committed and hardworking state agent I met in Vietnam. In addition to her twelve-hour workday, Hạnh frequently found herself on overnight trips to outlying regions far from the provincial capital, where she engaged in training activities aimed at preparing commune veterinarians for livestock disease outbreaks.

I also spent several weeks with district-level veterinarians as they implemented mass-vaccination measures in the region. Together we pushed motorbikes over muddy paddies, hopped on and off the boats and rafts traversing delta canals, encountered unruly farmers and infected flocks, labored under the tropical sun and heaving storms, skipped afternoon siestas, and fought against the most stubborn actors of all—ducks who battled against our grasping hands and probing needles. Working with veterinarians demonstrated the multiple demands placed on state agents in a landscape of pandemic risk. These veterinarians struggled with the task of carrying out HPAI control measures amid their other responsibilities, all while attempting to gain the trust of farmers who have long been suspicious of government.

At each of these sites I learned that bird flu interventions are embedded in distinct yet entangled public health, livestock production, and biomedical sectors, all of which feature their own locally specific sets of moral obligations, interpersonal relations, and commercial transactions. Working with multinational experts as well as farmers and state vets exposed how inadequate it would be to assume that pandemic policies are developed by global scientific experts working from technoscientific hubs, and then simply rolled out in outbreak areas. Instead, my research revealed how pandemic interventions are made *and remade* on the ground, in state policy arenas and in the everyday labor of livestock care.

Epicenter of Infection

How did Vietnam, a small nation in the corner of Southeast Asia, become a center of avian flu infection and intervention? Epidemiologists suggest that as migratory birds fly over East and Southeast Asia, they transmit less pathogenic, "wild" forms of the bird flu virus to domesticated flocks, which then go on to mutate into highly pathogenic strains (Gauthier-Clerc, Lebarbenchon, and Thomas 2007). These mutations are thought to happen more easily in places where patterns of livestock production bring animals into closer and more frequent contact with one another, other domesticated species, and humans. Vietnam offers both of these conditions of pandemic possibility.

Over the last four decades, Vietnamese livestock production has undergone substantial changes as political-economic developments transform the ways humans interact with rural landscapes and their inhabitants. After the fall of Saigon and the reunification of Vietnam in 1975, the Communist central government intensified moves to collectivize agriculture, seize ownership over industry and finance, and maintain state control over domestic markets. These policies were carried out against widespread mortal and environmental destruction wrought by thirty years of protracted war, devastating trade embargoes, and regional hostilities exacerbated by the unification of North and

South Vietnam. By the end of the first decade of national independence, the Vietnamese economy featured hyperinflation, food shortages, a large deficit, and growing labor unrest (Harvie 1997). In response to these trends, and following nascent market formation processes that started in the late 1970s, the central government installed a series of *đổi mới* economic reforms beginning in 1986. Signaling a "turn to the new," these reforms reduced the state's presence in economic activities: private industry grew, foreign investors began influencing the domestic market, and agricultural policy makers set their sights on export markets (Pritchett 1993). Guided by farm decollectivization, price liberalization, and increased opportunities for land use and ownership, Vietnam saw significant gains in agricultural production. The country went from a rice importer in 1988 to a rice exporter in the following year, and by the early 1990s Vietnam was the second largest rice exporter in the world (Dollar 1998). The growth of a substantial export industry in coffee, seafood, rubber, cashews, and pepper has added to positive assessments of Vietnam's market-led development.

These macro-level shifts have affected citizens' daily lives and their consumption patterns. Vietnam's transition to a socialist-oriented market economy has seen gross domestic product grow at steady rates for nearly four decades (World Bank 2018; Justino, Litchfield, and Pham 2008), and a recent forecast by PricewaterhouseCoopers notes that the country may have the fastest-growing economy in the world (PricewaterhouseCoopers 2017). The rising incomes associated with this growth have created a demand for protein-rich meats such as chicken and duck. Poultry production and consumption have increased at steady rates since the early 1990s as domestic food demand continues to shift away from rice toward livestock products (McLeod et al. 2006, 4). As global trade brings new foodstuffs into circulation, particularly in urban areas, daily meals that were once composed of rice and vegetables (with the occasional addition of fish) have been augmented with chicken, pork, and even beef. At the same time, Kentucky Fried Chicken, Loteria, and other multinational corporate food vendors have been proliferating in urban centers, stimulating appetites for meat-centric meals. Poultry consumption was reaching unprecedented levels prior to the bird flu outbreaks. Between 1998 and 2003, poultry consumption in Ho Chi Minh City alone increased by more than 100 percent, and on a national scale chicken production rose an average of 8.9 percent from 2001 to 2005 (Hong Hanh, Burgos, and Roland-Holst 2007, 8).

Such transformations in livestock production and consumption are not unique to Vietnam. Across Asia, chicken farming has expanded nearly 4.5 percent a year from 2000 to 2012 (Shah 2016). Even further afield, increases in population, urbanization, and income in Egypt, Nigeria, Brazil, and India have also been fueling demand for meat and milk products, provoking small-scale producers to intensify their participation in animal markets. Agricultural experts have posited a worldwide "Livestock Revolution," and have suggested that growing economies, particularly in Asia, will come to dictate the contours of global livestock markets by 2025 (Delgado, Rosegrant, and Meijer 2002).

In Vietnam, however, the increased demand for poultry products has occurred against the backdrop of a shrinking agricultural economy. As the country turns to light manufacturing and the service sector as drivers of economic growth, large-scale, agro-industrial and commercial poultry operations have grown slowly. This has left the burden of meeting consumer demand to small-scale poultry producers who continue to dominate national output, but whose dwindling landholdings cannot accommodate growing stocks of birds (Otte 2007). Intensified production has resulted in poultry densities previously unknown in the countryside. More productive commercial breeds have gained a foothold in household farms and in local and regional markets where they often mix with native flocks without regard to the origin or destination of the animals. Furthermore, as livestock agriculture intensifies, it becomes increasingly reliant on pharmaceuticals. The increased use of hormones, steroids, and other growth and reproductive therapies is part of a globalized trend toward micromanaging every stage of the livestock production process—from conception to consumption—in order to maximize profit. These drugs are contributing to the creation of biologically weak animals, animals who cannot endure a gesture, a pet, or even a kind word from humans without risking miscarriage, injury, or death (Blanchette 2018). In Vietnam, antibiotics, vaccines, and antivirals have become mainstays in a largely unregulated pharmaceutical market, where they find their way into poultry not only through the hands of state veterinarians like those I worked with in Đồng Tháp, but also through the hands of untrained farmers and semi-trained para-veterinary professionals. Antibiotic resistance has become commonplace in poultry flocks, many of which have only been partially vaccinated for major infections, thereby making them doubly vulnerable to disease (Fermet-Quinet, Edan, and Stratton 2010).

These vulnerabilities are then carried off the farm as farmers like Thủy and Trí multiply their market contacts beyond village gates and into neighboring districts, provinces, and cities where livestock fetches a higher price. Such trends mean that ducks and chickens travel along increasingly diversified market chains—on the bicycles, boats, and motorbikes of independent traders and farmers themselves, or in the trucks of certified poultry transporters to major wholesale markets as well as the thousands of retail wet markets and street vendors across urban and peri-urban areas. Markets, in turn, serve as meeting grounds for people, poultry, and pathogens. As consumers swap cash for fowl, poultry swap microbes and viruses with one another , as well as with other animals for sale. In short, increased production, movement, and sale of poultry have taken place in informally organized, densely populated, and ecologically unstable settings.

Such livestock market patterns have, according to some experts, opened up new and dangerous disease ecologies, and as soon as the flu outbreaks in northern Vietnam were linked to the H5N1 virus, poultry farmers began to suffer. Officials and volunteers began "bird hunting" in villages, destroying chickens and ducks that were either offered up by or forced out of farmers' hands (Vo 2004). For several weeks, the newly formed National Steering Committee on Human and Avian Influenza prohibited the production, slaughter, and consumption of poultry in outbreak areas, and strictly regulated these activities in the rest of the country. Between 2003 and 2005, nearly sixty million poultry died or were slaughtered as a result of bird flu infections, and the government estimated losses of over two hundred million U.S. dollars in the first year alone. These losses were most strongly felt among small-scale farmers who constituted nearly two-thirds of poultry production (Morris et al. 2005).[4]

One Health Governance

The scale of human, animal, and economic losses to avian flu, combined with threats of the virus's global spread, has made Vietnam a locus for multinational and nongovernmental interventions against the disease, and the country receives the highest per-capita amount of foreign avian flu aid of any nation (Vu 2009). Thirteen bilateral donor countries, several multi-donor trust funds, multilateral donors such as the World Bank and the Asian Development Bank, and regional organizations such as ASEAN and APEC have contributed over two hundred million US dollars for pandemic flu management in Vietnam. In addition, a host of bilateral and multinational organizations, including the United Nations Food and Agricultural Organization (FAO), the World Health Organization (WHO), the World Organization for Animal Health (OIE), and the Centers for Disease Control and Prevention (CDC), have provided sustained technical support for avian flu control. Added to the mix are more than twenty-five international, nongovernmental, nonprofit, and humanitarian organizations that together have mobilized vast human resources to address the disease (National Steering Committee on Human and Avian Influenza 2006a).

The multinational organizations assembling around bird flu in Vietnam are not only confronting unstable and shifting disease ecologies; they are also working within a transforming national health care system. Over the last three decades, economic reforms have altered Vietnam's onetime state monopoly on the provision of health services.[5] Đổi mới renovations have introduced a series of health policies that include legalizing private medical practice, privatizing pharmaceutical production and sale, and introducing fees in public medical facilities. The number of registered and unregistered private practitioners has catapulted, having exceeded two thousand by the mid-1990s (Smithson 1993), pharmacies have begun to appear on nearly every city street and have become increasingly prevalent in rural communes (Craig 2002). Vietnam's universal health care has shifted toward an unregulated, mixed private-public system in which more and more citizens are choosing self-treatment over public health services (Sepheri and Akram-Lodhi 2005, 137). Organizations like the World Bank, USAID, and the WHO are encouraging further reductions in the state financing of health services. This has transferred the costs of disease control to citizens, and has organized the provision of health care around market principles of cost-effectiveness (Keevers, Treleaven, and Sykes 2008).

Shifts in Vietnam's public health system have strained state-employed health workers. While Hạnh, the intrepid veterinarian I worked with in Đồng Tháp, was unique among her peers in choosing government work, her husband and her college classmates had all taken up veterinary positions at commercial feed companies. As their support from the central government has diminished, full-time government health employees have begun to supplement their incomes through part-time private practice. Fewer and fewer human and animal health workers look for work in the public sector, preferring to bolster their incomes through entrepreneurial endeavors or by joining up with private or multinational veterinary and human health agencies. Additionally, foreign donors have become indispensable financiers of Vietnam's public health systems, and citizens increasingly seek health care from nonstate agencies or private providers (Smithson 1993). The diversity of health donors and providers has made it difficult for the government to coordinate funds and services within a coherent health investment plan. Since the mid-1990s analysts have been calling for Vietnam to develop a more comprehensible health care system (Chen and Hiebert 1994, 15).

Such trends have been consequential to globalized bird flu management.

As Theresa MacPhail (2014a) explains, global health is like a virus: it does not exist without host institutions and local milieus, and it cannot survive without constantly adapting to them. Vietnam's particular strain of global health is one in which the nation-state appears front and center. Since the onset of H5N1 outbreaks in 2004, the Vietnamese government has been concerned with establishing a commanding presence in bird flu management. Keen to exercise influence on bird flu policies and practices, Communist Party officials have systematically brought nongovernmental organizations and multinational donors into the fold of a centralized governing structure. Their first move was to create the National Steering Committee on Human and Avian Influenza (NSCAI) under the codirection of the Ministry of Health and Ministry of Agriculture and Rural Development. Through the NSCAI framework, these government bodies exercise executive power over all avian flu financing and programming: they set national avian flu agendas, distribute funds and personnel across institutions, and monitor project activities (National Steering Committee on Human and Avian Influenza 2006a). In 2006, the NSCAI established Government–UN Joint Program on Avian and Human Pandemic Influenza to "harmonize" and streamline the funding and activities of government agencies, the United Nations, bilateral and multilateral donors, and NGOs. As part of the harmonization process, on-the-ground bird flu collaborations are designed and carried out in formalized partnerships between state and non-state agencies. This effectively means that the state has inserted government health workers in all bird flu-related activities. As one UN avian flu advisor explained, "The [Communist] Party is brilliant. It's using multinational organizations *to strengthen* its influence."[6]

Such harmonization is fueled by a history of Vietnam's centrist state government dictating the terms of global integration since *đổi mới* (Porter 1993). In a review of rural development projects, researchers David Craig and Doug Porter conclude that the government is careful to coordinate foreign donors and consultancies under its own planning ambits through extensive partnerships and networking processes (Craig and Porter 2006, 128). Supranational health officials favor this sort of state involvement because it falls in line with efforts to promote sustainable, long-term health programming in which national governments take leadership roles in addressing health problems. The United Nations' senior coordinator for avian flu put it this way: "You don't maintain control over this disease unless there is regular top-level direction from a senior committed political figure that wants to be sure the necessary activities are being undertaken" (McKenna 2006). In sum, Vietnam's experience suggests that global health is not necessarily a juggernaut of multinational governance eroding state institutions; that multinational organizations do not always constitute a "republic of NGOs" (Farmer 2011) or an "unruly mélange" of actors pursuing different interests (Buse and Walt 1997). There are conflict and competition among different health organizations addressing bird flu, but these organizations nevertheless operate under broadly agreed upon, state-defined objectives and chains of command.

Vietnam's unique trajectory of bird flu emergence and governance reveals two important points. First, the country's historically, economically, and culturally specific arrangements of humans, animals, and environments have fostered the conditions for bird flu's global reappearance and spread. Second, the country's central government is doing much to shape the trajectory of global pandemic programming, in keeping with its unique political history and its agenda for international integration. This means that the hegemony of the state and the hegemony of multinational institutions exist in productive tension with each other regarding bird flu governance. Power and influence flow in multiple directions. Attentive to these dynamics, I understand global health *as a collection of situated, intersecting practices and perspectives that local, state, and multinational actors use to address problems affecting worldwide populations.* I suggest that if we look carefully at these different practices and perspectives, and explore how they come together in the everyday work of bird flu governance, we will come to see many different articulations of "global" health.

The story of bird flu in Vietnam is therefore a story about multinational actors interacting with and transforming state institutions amid worldwide neoliberal health reforms. It is a story about states asserting themselves in global health orders, through the everyday activities of government agents who work both with and against multinational organizations in the name of national sovereignty and community well-being. It is a story about how historically and culturally specific poultry rearing practices both affect, and are affected by, global market formations and the shifting contours of livestock production worldwide. By locating the pandemic threat in Vietnam, I argue that no matter how global the H5N1 virus is, and no matter how deterritorialized the mechanisms for addressing it may be, bird flu emerges at particular moments and in particular places. Place matters in global health.

Place matters in global health, but so do animals. It is therefore curious that nonhuman animals are absent in much of the literature on pandemic flu, which often focuses on the logics, institutions, and practices aimed at preventing outbreaks in humans. In this book I take a different tact. I proceed from a recognition that bird flu is not just pushing the purview of public health beyond the nation-state; it is also pushing the purview of public health beyond the human. Just as H5N1 was making its presence felt around the world, a group of international health experts gathered in New York City to address growing concerns about *zoonoses*, or diseases passed between human and nonhuman animals. They concluded that these infections are best addressed through a unified approach that brings human and nonhuman animal health together: One Health (Cook, Karesh, and Osofsky 2009).[7] The One Health movement has created new collaborations among crucial global players in human and animal health,[8] and in outbreak areas like Vietnam these collaborations manifest in on-the-ground interventions that bring veterinarians, biologists, public health workers, and even national security experts together to tackle the complex, and sometimes pathogenic, interconnections between species.

Yet, despite its ambitious goals and interdisciplinary interventions, so far One Health is failing to address interspecies interconnections in ways that prevent infection (Smith, Taylor, and Kingsley 2015). Even in Vietnam, where endless resources have been used to control bird flu, the H5N1 virus has become endemic, or enzootic, which means that it is constantly circulating among domestic poultry. How has this happened? One explanation is that One Health interventions are overly technoscientific and targeted. Poultry vaccine measures and on-the-farm hygiene inputs might obstruct virus transmission routes, but they do not address the social, historical, and political-economic conditions that allow these transmission routes to form in the first place. That is, they do not address the spatial limitations that compel farmers like Trí and Thủy to invest in high-density flocks, or the market fluctuations that incite them to transport their birds across far distances in search of better prices. Similarly, biosecure agro-industrial zones may effectively separate poultry from people, but they do not account for the familial ties and obligations that prevent farmers from moving their flocks away from densely populated natal villages. Finally, interventions that limit poultry movements and standardize their breeding and feeding regimens do not consider how culturally situated farming practices associate healthy poultry with local varieties and free-ranging behaviors.

In other words, One Health governance fails to properly account for the conditions under which farmers and fowl actually live. This book is my attempt to account for those conditions. I describe the biological, cultural, and economic relations among people and poultry in a context where pandemic control programs are generating novel strategies for governing human and nonhuman animal life. Crucially, throughout this account, I draw attention to the fact that poultry are life forms as well as livestock—market laborers and commodities. This means that any disease-control strategy targeting poultry must be understood and evaluated as both a public health *and* an economic intervention.

Early on, the Vietnamese government recognized the economic risks and opportunities of One Health programming for bird flu, and it developed a national program that explicitly linked disease control to agro-economic development. A primary objective of Vietnam's bird flu policy has been to restructure domestic poultry production in order to align it with industrial, commercial standards. According to the NSCAI Integrated National Plan for Avian Influenza Control and Human Pandemic Preparedness and Response 2006–10:

> The goal of the government's Strategy for Agriculture and Rural Development 2001–2010 is to restructure the agricultural sector to become more competitive and demand-driven. As part of this strategy, [the Ministry of Agriculture and Rural Development] has the long-term aim to *industrialize* poultry farming, slaughtering and processing. This objective has implications for HPAI control, including opportunities to improve bio-security in production, and control the poultry marketing chain (National Steering Committee on Human and Avian Influenza 2006c, vi–vii, emphasis added).

The purposeful linking of biosecurity and poultry-sector industrialization is not unique to Vietnam. It corresponds with an ongoing effort by the World Organization for Animal Health (OIE) and the UN Food and Agriculture Organization (FAO) to develop biosafety and security standards for global livestock markets (World Organization for Animal Health 2015). At a more local level, these standardizing processes work in tandem with a Vietnamese governmental strategy to prepare domestic poultry production for eventual export. As a global health cum national economic strategy, restructuring limits flu infection while at the same time propelling Vietnamese poultry into standardized, industrial, and market-ready commodity chains, where it could eventually join rice, shrimp, and cashews as part of a growing bundle of Vietnamese exports.[9]

In restructuring Vietnamese livestock economies, the country's avian flu strategy is also redefining the subjects and outcomes of public health intervention. Restructuring activities conceive of poultry as both targets and tools of disease control. But only certain kinds of poultry combat disease in this health model: *industrial, commercial* breeds that differ in quality and kind from native fowl in Vietnam. Restructuring also conceives of poultry farmers as the targets and tools of disease control. But again, only certain kinds of farmers: *industrial, commercial* cultivators who engage in contractual relations with corporations or state farms and agree to abide by commercial standards of production. But by delineating industrial fowl and farmers as the subjects and beneficiaries of health intervention, restructuring also promises to erode traditional free-ranging farming practices, whereby small farmers independently raise native or hybrid breeds for personal consumption and local market sales. Poultry sector restructuring will therefore push millions of fowl and farmers out of the livestock economy altogether, and this in a country where over 80 percent of rural dwellers engage in some form of poultry production for basic subsistence, for supplementary income, or as a primary wage-earning activity.

The NSCAI recognizes the negative economic implications of this governing strategy for small farmers and has made countless statements to the effect that restructuring must proceed with an eye toward preserving farmers' livelihoods. But apart from this nod to equity, little attention has been paid to the biological, social, and political consequences of poultry sector restructuring in communities where poultry is woven into kin-based agricultural production systems, where it figures centrally in ritual practice, and where it serves as a symbol for rural wealth and health. This is true not only for Vietnam, but also for other countries where H5N1 is prevalent, and where small-scale, household farms capture a large portion of the poultry market (Hinchliffe and Bingham 2008; Lowe 2010; Fearnley 2018).

In short, One Health governance for H5N1 is transforming the kinds of life worth living, and the kinds of lifestyles and livelihoods worth protecting—in Vietnam and beyond. Understanding these transformations requires foregrounding not just animals, but also markets, property, and exchange relations—economies—in pandemic planning. It also requires examining pandemics in terms of inequality and not just risk or preparedness. This is a less frequently told story of pandemics, but it is one that begs to be told in an era of One Health exhortations that encourage integrating animals into global health without fully addressing the specific economies within which animals and their pathogens circulate.

Multispecies Exchange Relations

To more fully account for the economies in which One Health governance operates, I detail the multispecies exchange relationships that surface in the daily work of bird flu prevention and control. Exchange relationships are everywhere in bird flu interventions, particularly in the poultry economies that suffer losses from viral outbreaks. The relationships here are unsettled. Poultry are first and foremost domesticated animals, whose very existence is

a result of purposeful biotechnological manipulation, and whose life trajectories are dictated by efforts to sustain human life and livelihoods. But such
efforts do not always work, and as virus hosts and vectors, poultry indicate
biological forces beyond human control—forces that humans must contend
with and adapt to in order to survive. H5N1 thus challenges popular understandings of domestication as a unilinear process in which human beings
dominate nature. To fully capture this disease and its implications, I require
an approach that attends not only to relations of hierarchy and control, but
also to instances of mutual transformation and becoming, in which humans
and nonhumans shape each other's conditions of existence (Haraway 2007;
Lien 2015).

Multispecies ethnography is a mode of investigation that focuses attention on culturally and historically specific relationships between species, and
explores how those relationships shape social worlds (Kirksey and Helmreich 2010). With its interest in understanding nonhumans as both biological and social actors, multispecies ethnography offers a fruitful framework
for exploring bird flu in outbreak locations like Vietnam, where relations
between species not only foster pandemic threats, but also structure efforts
to contain them (Lowe 2010; Porter 2013). My aim in research and writing
has been to analytically foreground people-poultry-pathogen relationships
in order to give a fuller picture of disease-control processes, rather than a
more limited account that primarily addresses human actors. Practically
speaking, this meant placing myself near poultry and the people living closest to them, paying close attention to (and sometimes sharing in) exchanges
between species—particularly those that seemed relevant to disease control.
Importantly, this approach did not mean that people, poultry, and pathogens
are equal actors in the worlds I observed or have written about. Interspecies
exchanges in livestock economies are often instrumental, hierarchical, and
violent. We must not forget that poultry are made to live and die in the service of human appetites.

And yet, just because poultry are domesticated, commoditized, and con-
sumed does not mean they are inconsequential social actors. Livestock animals have long played a critical role in the history of capitalist formations
(Horowitz 2004; Ritvo 1987; Shukin 2009),[10] and anthropologists have been
concerned with documenting this role in a variety of social and cultural settings (Blanchette 2015; Comaroff and Comaroff 1990; Hutchinson 1996; Lien
2015; Pachirat 2013). Sarah Franklin's genealogical study of sheep provides an
exemplary model. She shows that as sheep production drove the development
of British agriculture and industry, it transformed landscapes and displaced
peoples, and helped justify processes of empire building. Sheep have con-

tinued to shape economic and social life in Britain and beyond. Innovative sheep breeding techniques are driving developments in global biotechnology, generating new industries and life forms that challenge long-held ideas about kinship, sex, and the integrity of species (remember Dolly the cloned sheep). By treating sheep as animal *and* capital, life *and* stock, Franklin is able to show how they embody complex and evolving economic, national, and biological relationships. These relationships shape ideas about how to live, but they also result in displacement, dispossession, and death (2007, 153–54).

Taking a similar approach, in this book I also trace the complex and ever-evolving relations between animal and capital, life and stock. Writing from the vantage point of Vietnam, an epicenter of pandemic risk, I focus attention on the ways in which people-poultry relations shape rural livelihoods, national economies, and transnational relations in a time of uncertainty and danger. My goal is to show how these multispecies relations are radically transforming, as One Health governance sparks new calculations about how best to cultivate and control livestock. Focusing on exchange relations in livestock economies allows me to view how farmers and fowl *push against* the kinds of displacements and dispossessions that come along with poultry sector restructuring for flu control. Farmers' everyday exchanges with chickens and ducks—in households, on farms, and in markets—reveal that there are other meanings and values at play in Vietnamese livestock economies, those that do not so easily equate poultry with their commercial function. Bird flu interventions thus encounter complications in communities where immunity and profit are weighed against other estimations of livestock value.

But poultry are not the only consequential nonhumans in this story. Alongside the economies suffering losses from virus outbreaks are those poised to profit from them. These are biomedical economies, where the primary targets and tools of flu intervention are viruses and the commodities developed from them. More and more, organic life forms are becoming sources of raw materials, labor, and value in the bioeconomy (Waldby and Mitchell 2006; Parry 2004; Hayden 2003). Viruses are no exception, and since the bird flu outbreaks, vaccine and antiviral manufacturers have been scrambling to develop H5N1 samples into marketable therapies. Biomedical start-ups and Big Pharma alike have touted revolutionary approaches to pandemic flu, including aerosol vaccines, nano-based therapeutics, and handheld diagnostic devices.

Viruses are valuable. But when they appear in therapies with public health applications, they raise ethical questions about the equitable distribution of health resources in the event of a pandemic. Bird flu in particular has raised questions about who can claim ownership over pandemic viruses, which appear in one place but can potentially spread everywhere. The disease has also sparked debates about who can have access to costly vaccines and antivirals in a global health arena where life and health are considered basic human rights (Hinterberger and Porter 2015; Lezaun and Montgomery 2015). These are systemic questions about the transnational appropriation and exchange of viruses and virus-derived therapies. But they also surface in on-the-ground interventions, for instance in farmers' struggles over scarce supplies of state-subsidized vaccines. At different scales, virus exchange relations embody tensions between the public ethos of global public health and the proprietary devices of biomedicine.

Viruses, in fact, are fundamentally relational entities. These "quasi-species" (Lowe 2010) are never autonomous; they can only truly live or function within the cells of a host. In the process of infection, viruses draw organisms together through shared histories, spaces, and bodily substances—through exchanges. Erin Koch (2013) put it best when she said that microbes form an integral part of the social fabric. On this view, scholars in anthropology and science studies have recently challenged ideas about viruses as purely parasitic and destructive external agents (MacPhail 2004; Cohen 2011; Greenhough 2012; Serres 2007) and have instead traced both the positive and negative effects of human-microbial intermingling (Paxson 2008, 2012; Lorimer 2018, 2017; Wolf-Meyer 2017). Expanding on this scholarship, I contend that it is important to trace how the effects of microbial exchange relations are unequally distributed across different communities of humans living with animals. That is, I want to show how viruses shape different worlds differently, and to think about what this means for *One* Health.

Taken together, this multispecies analysis takes poultry and pathogens as part of the social fabric, and it traces the everyday exchanges in which these life forms become productive forces for markets while simultaneously engaging in a variety of consequential relations with humans. This approach is attentive to but slightly athwart the kinds of analyses associated with the ontological turn in anthropology. Drawing on a long-standing interest in indigenous worldviews and the ways that nonhuman beings achieve personhood (Hallowell 1992; Ingold 1980, 1988; Bulmer 1973), these pathbreaking accounts posit that subjects, nature, and even reality are multiple and relative (Kohn 2013; Vivieros de Castro 2004; Willerslev 2004). I am also interested in suspending assumptions about species differences and social hierarchies and in rejecting notions about the integrity and the ascendancy of the human that are often taken for granted. This work is critical for developing a more inclusive politics that challenges the separation of nature and culture, and that advances nonhumans as significant social and political actors

(Povinelli 1995; Cadena 2015; Muñoz 2015; Nadasdy 2003, 2007; Hartigan 2014). At the same time, however, I remain attentive to violence and inequality, displacement and dispossession that animate livestock economies. This means providing a fine-grained account of the uneven and shifting distribution of agency among humans and nonhumans in bird flu governance, and exposing relentless efforts to prioritize certain life forms and lifeways over others (Ogden, Hall, and Tanita 2013, 13). As Juno Parrenas (2015) suggests, to write within the ontological turn is "not to ignore imposed hierarchies. . . . Rather, we need to be attuned to multiple hierarchies and open to surprises."

This is a story, then, of global relations of power and inequality seen through the lens of multispecies exchange relations—between viruses and hosts; farmers and fowl; commercial and noncommercial actors; health workers and citizens; and state agents, scientists, and pharmaceutical developers. It is a story of how these exchanges generate new life forms and new ways of living with others in a context of pandemic risk. To be sure, the exchanges viewed here are uneven, as different actors jockey for position in Vietnam's emergent One Health order. But these exchanges are also unsettled and transformative, as One Health interventions create new possibilities for poultry production and consumption, alter existing health institutions and practices, and introduce new substances and sentiments into biomedical and livestock economies. In other words, these exchanges are experimental.

Experiment

A central argument of this book is that One Health interventions are best understood as a series of experiments in governing multispecies relations. Building on scholarship in anthropology and science and technology studies, I see experiments as much more than instruments for testing hypotheses under controlled conditions.[11] Hans-Jorg Rheinberger (1997) famously describes experiments as systems, which draw together different ideas, organisms, and practices in order to address problems and imagine futures. Experimental systems are ordered yet heterogeneous; components in the system respond to experimental conditions in ways that cannot always be anticipated or controlled. For Rheinberger, such built-in uncertainty is what allows experiments to produce valid knowledge.

Pushing the concept of experiment further, critics of public health remind us that experiments are as much about intervening and controlling as they are about imagining and investigating. Anthropologist and physician Vinh-Kim Nguyen (2009) coins the term "experimentality" to describe the relationship between experiment and governmentality (the strategies used to control populations). Looking at West African HIV programs, he shows how state and non-state organizations carry out experiments that generate knowledge *through* the act of intervening in affected populations. These experiments are often the only sources of health care available, which means that disease sufferers must conform to experimental conditions in order to survive.

Life itself is therefore at stake in global health experiments. Michelle Murphy elucidates this fact in ways that have helped me think through bird flu control in Vietnam. Murphy describes how, during the period of the Cold War and decolonization, social and biological scientists sought to *economize life* by calculating which lives were worth living and sustaining, which lives were worthy of investment, and which lives were not worth being born (2017, 6). Experiments to govern reproduction proliferated, particularly in the postcolonial Global South, where they shaped bodily practices as well as desires for better futures. Drawing from Nguyen, Murphy suggests that these experiments comprised a kind of governmentality in the postcolony—they reached beyond the lab, the clinic, and even the field site to households, markets, and villages where they fostered new forms of expertise and social relations (2017, 79). Experiments, then, are exercises in valuing life, determining life chances, and fashioning ways of life.

I define One Health experiments as *activities that bring different organisms, ideas, technologies, and practices together in order to produce knowledge about life forms while simultaneously valuing and transforming them.* Experiments are oriented toward the present and the future; they seek to address problems in the here and now in order to engender something different down the line. This means that experiments can take place in sites not usually associated with scientific or even public health practice—places where real world problems surface, and where a variety of actors and interests can weigh in on their solutions. This definition captures both the exploratory and the normative dimensions of One Health experiments, or how they assert particular agendas, values, and inequalities even as they explore the unknown and uncertain.

In the pages that follow, I introduce a cadre of experts from multinational, state, and nongovernmental organizations. Trained in public health, veterinary medicine, virology, and social science, these experts engage in experimental activities that promote certain life forms and lifestyles over others, all as part of an imagined future free from infectious poultry and its unruly producers. The "real world experiments" (Biesel 2015, 293) they pursue expand beyond traditional sites of scientific practice and reach into households, farms, markets, and even individual bodies. Critically, as they bleed into their broader social milieu, these experiments become sites of negotiation and conflict as different actors (human and otherwise) pursue different interests.

Another key argument of this book is that One Health experiments generate negotiation and conflict because they attempt to bridge the aims of global public health with those of domestic livestock production. This means that flu experiments do not just govern life; they also commoditize it. In her account of reproductive governance, Michelle Murphy distinguishes between economizing and commoditizing life: economizing life manages surplus life for nations (designating which lives and lifestyles are valuable and therefore worth living), while commoditizing life generates surplus value for markets (turning life forms into consumable products). Economizing and commoditizing exist alongside one another, but for Murphy they are distinct. This distinction does not hold in One Health governance. Bird flu experiments target people *and* poultry, which are both life forms and commodities—life and stock. Bird flu experiments designate which human and animal lives should be invested in or disinvested from, to optimize human health and the national economy, but this process always includes governing the human and nonhuman labor that creates market commodities. In more-than-human health governance, the value of human life is always articulated alongside the value of nonhuman animal life as creature-commodities. Understanding One Health experiments therefore requires examining the stakes and consequences for different actors when bird flu is framed differently—by global health experts as a threat to humans, by state leaders as a threat to national economies, and by farmers as a threat to poultry, rural livelihoods, and market relationships.

Governance—multispecies exchange relations—experiments. These braided concepts are critical for understanding the uneven socioeconomic relations, and uneven valuations of life that shape what is and what is not possible for bird flu control at various times and places, and on various scales. They provide an analytical lens through which to view the more-than-human interactions that inform, resist, and restructure One Health on the ground. And they point to interwoven practices of controlling, valuing, and commoditizing life, practices belying any claim that One Health is just about health.

Tracing the experimental, multispecies exchange relations that surface in bird flu control programs allows me to expose and push against what I have come to see as the key limitation of One Health governance: an impoverished and singular way of classifying the world. For all its talk of human-animal interfaces and the unity of the world's creatures, One Health proceeds from the position that disease agents and their hosts are fundamentally separate entities whose bodies can be manipulated, and whose interactions can be mapped and managed, for the purposes of infection control. I argue that this idea not only fails to capture the ways that people actually live with poultry and pathogens in Vietnam (and elsewhere), but that it also engenders a series of betrayals. Commercializing poultry production in the name of global health and national economic development betrays the kin-based livelihood activities and land use practices from which poultry producers like Thủy and Trí derive meaning and value. The breed distinctions, uniform feed inputs, and standardized farmer-fowl interactions that are so common to commercial poultry production betray culturally significant relationships between species that have long been based on shared spaces and freedom of movement. Circumscribing heterogeneous poultry markets into commercialized industrial value chains betrays farmers' hard-won ability to move in and out of income generating activities in late-socialist Vietnam by cultivating a variety of life forms for a variety of trading partners.

In short, One Health betrays the world-making activities of Vietnamese farmers and fowl. This betrayal is not limited to Vietnam. Bird flu, swine flu, MERS, Ebola, rabies, monkey pox, HIV, dengue, all of these diseases have incited interventions that seek to conquer viral risks by separating viruses from hosts and vectors, and by separating hosts from one another—this despite the fact that these bodily distinctions and separations have proven time and time again impossible to uphold.[12] As I write these words, news is spreading about a new WHO strategy to prepare for an unknown but looming zoonotic "Disease X" (R. J. 2018). That a zoonotic pandemic still looms today, over a decade since H5N1 reemerged on the world scene, suggests that we need new ideas and new tools for living and living well with others.

Ethnography can provide these ideas and tools. The exchanges between people, poultry, and pathogens that I chart throughout this book open up space for considering alternative classifications of the world. The exchanges that occur on and off the farm do not always stem from efforts to establish and maintain boundaries between species, or efforts to meet commercial standards of productivity and profit. They show that there are ways of living with others that do not identify zoonoses as the primary risk to multispecies health and well-being. Instead, they signal another possibility: that the homogenization of poultry commodities and the overregulation of poultry markets might be a graver threat to life and livelihoods.

In the chapters that follow, I will show that Vietnamese farmers actually already *live* a more-than-human health; they set their sights beyond species divisions, and beyond biology, to cultivate a variety of modes to manage life, livestock, and livelihoods. Yet, these multiple orientations to life and stock, and these multiple forms of control and care cannot be encapsulated in a decidedly singular One Health paradigm that largely acts in service of global livestock standardization. This is where my concept of experiment gains its practical power. Although experiments always include forms of violence and exclusion, insofar as they aim to make something different happen, they hold open possibilities for refusal, and for imagining a different politics of life (Murphy 2017, 80, 144). As George Marcus and Michael Fischer write, we can see experiment as a critique that pushes the envelope of conventional understandings *and* as a practical mode of intervening in and changing the world (Marcus and Fischer 1999, xxxii). My task in this book is to consider the implications of the multispecies world-making activities I encountered in Vietnam, and to take them seriously as viable possibilities for living with others in a pandemic age. In doing so, my goal is not simply to criticize One Health, but rather to reimagine what health could look like in spaces where different life forms are brought together in unanticipated and deliberately experimental ways. This book, then, multiplies the world.

Plan of the Book

Each chapter in this book describes a particular avian flu experiment and situates it in the broader economies in which it surfaces. I describe the people, poultry, and pathogens caught up in the experiment, and trace the exchange relationships that connect them to one another and to the larger One Health ecology. Interspersed through the chapters are short interludes that detail the historical, cultural, and symbolic relations between people and poultry in Vietnam. The insights I offer here are partial, but when taken together they illuminate the locally specific, experimental exchanges that actually comprise One Health governance.

Chapter 1, "Experimental Entrepreneurs," examines two biosecurity experiments to cultivate infection-free, economically productive poultry subpopulations. The first experiment introduces "model ducks" by applying biosecurity containment principles to free-ranging farms in the Mekong Delta. The second experiment cultivates "Naturally Vietnam" chickens and utilizes traditional backyard farming methods to thwart exposure to pathogens. I show that both experiments invest in new, flu-free life forms/commodities, each of which requires farmers to transform their ways of life by altering their labor practices and culturally situated exchange relations with poultry. I further reflect on how these animals reveal different ideas about the role of poultry in agricultural ecologies and economies, and different understandings of the role of commercial market standards in governing human health subjects. I conclude that in a global health landscape characterized by increasingly market-oriented health programming, biosecurity experiments signal a nascent model of disease control, which conceives of at-risk populations less as vulnerable subjects and more as economically productive entrepreneurs.

Chapter 2, "Enumerating Immunity," considers mass poultry vaccination, which was initially conceived as a short-term measure to reduce the amount of H5N1 virus in Vietnamese poultry populations. My aim here is to trace H5N1 vaccines as they circulate in rural duck and chicken producing communities. I trace the quotidian activities of veterinary professionals in Đồng Tháp and Bắc Giang provinces in order to show that in a national context of scarce resources and the privatization of health services, state veterinarians distribute vaccine supplies in uneven and unreliable ways. This spotty exchange of resources prompts farmers to protect their flocks through other means (namely kin-based transactions), and in accordance with their own assessments of bird flu risks in relation to other biothreats. The exchanges between state agents, farmers, and fowl in vaccination campaigns suggest that quick-fix experiments to safeguard human populations through the inoculation of birds find little purchase in settings where bird flu inordinately affects poultry, and where policy makers, veterinarians, and farmers have different priorities surrounding the protection of life, livelihoods, and livestock.

Chapter 3, "Commerce and Containment," examines poultry market restrictions. Drawing on fieldwork in and around Hanoi and Ho Chi Minh City, I describe how market restrictions are driven by a government desire to commercialize and industrialize the poultry circulating in urban "hotspots." Yet, such strategies to keep viruses out of the urban areas portend significant losses to "rural," semi-commercial farmers who have long traveled to and from the city to exchange money and commodities. Market restrictions therefore expose value-laden efforts to simultaneously economize and commoditize life in Vietnam: they draw on existing social hierarchies in order to promote certain kinds of livestock commodities and certain kinds of livelihood practices, all the while placing limits on others. But as an experiment, market restrictions produce mixed results. I relay a series of stories to show how farmers negotiated their movements at Vietnam's rural-urban edges in order to uphold livestock ownership rights, kin-based production practices, and access to markets. When situated in a historical context of agricultural development failures, these farmers' maneuvers reveal how One Health planning exacerbates ongoing struggles between the state and citizens over the terms and trajectories of livestock production.

Chapter 4, "Marketing Morals," moves the analysis to endemic-phase experiments centered on information communications. I show how behavior change communications campaigns imagine and create desires for different futures by using social marketing techniques to "sell" healthy behaviors to citizens as health consumers. While this choice-based approach to health provision seems incompatible with a Vietnamese governing system centered on compulsory state directives, my observations show how health and development workers unite these distinct governing practices in inventive ways. By juxtaposing bird flu communications with critical readings of propaganda posters from Vietnam's revolutionary era, I argue that bird flu commercials, jingles, slogans, and merchandise draw on long-standing socialist mass mobilization devices to establish a market in healthy behaviors. Symbols of family responsibility, state stewardship, and livestock care, which the government has long used to discipline populations, find ideological purchase in this experiment. I further argue that behavior change communications expose a shift in Vietnam's health governance, from governing self-responsible citizens in the Communist era, to governing self-responsible consumers in the market socialist era. Taken together, this analysis illustrates the everyday practices through which the Vietnamese state interacts with global health orders, and it shows the locally specific intersection of health and economic logics in One Health.

The final analytical chapter, "How to Own a Virus," looks beyond Vietnam in order to examine virus surveillance, a far-reaching and anticipatory intervention to track viral mutations, inform containment strategies, and guide the development and distribution of pharmaceuticals worldwide. Virus surveillance rests on exchange relations whereby affected nations freely forward human and animal H5N1 viruses to global laboratories and pharmaceutical companies. My aim here is to probe the notion of "sharing" that drives these surveillance strategies, by examining recent moves to tether avian flu viruses to the nations from which they emerged. I show that while novel claims of ownership over *human* flu viruses have caused national and supranational actors to experiment with new global virus-sharing arrangements, similar arrangements have not emerged for *animal* viruses. These species-specific virus exchanges reveal that, for all the talk of species jumping and spillover, human and animal viruses live very different social lives. They travel through different bodies, different scientific networks, and different commodity markets where they obtain very different sorts of moral, biological, and commercial value. I contend that these unsynchronized exchange relations are worth attending to because they illustrate the diverse economic and ethical interests that undergird global health security, and because they express the human exceptionalism that pervades the One Health formations that explicitly aim to move beyond it.

I conclude by recapitulating the governance-multispecies exchange relations-experiment framework developed throughout the book. I argue that a multi-sited, more-than-human analysis of experimental exchange relations can teach us a lot about what One Health looks like on the ground, in everyday encounters between people, poultry, and pathogens. This framework reveals the heterogeneous and unstable intersections between global public health and livestock economies, and it exposes the uneven value of life at various sites of zoonoses management. I end with a prompt to open One Health up to multiple, experimental ways of living with nonhuman animals and environments. Taking my cue from the people and poultry that animate this ethnography, I consider how differently positioned social actors—both human and nonhuman—address the cascading risks and opportunities posed by bird flu. I further suggest that within their various strategies for living together we can both glimpse and foster more reflexive and inclusive health: one that transcends platitudes about the common good by addressing the inevitable fact that different lives matter more than others, and one that surpasses market limitations by cultivating more diverse relations of care and companionship between species.

Gà *Ta*, Our Chicken

Legend has it that a chicken played a decisive role in the formation of the Vietnamese nation. Ethnic Vietnamese (Kính) people trace their origins to a union between a dragon lord, Lạc Long Quân, and a fairy queen, Âu Cơ. After they married, the fairy queen laid a sack of eggs that hatched into one hundred human sons, the eldest of whom became the first Hùng king of Vietnam. He and his descendents ruled for nearly two thousand years until their kingdom came under pressure from Chinese leaders extending their empire south. Eventually, one leader pressed into the Vietnamese territory, dethroned the last of the Hùng kings, and installed himself as King An Dương of his newly founded kingdom, Âu Lạc (257–179 BCE). Most of what is known of King An Dương comes from legends, and one in particular tells of his thwarted attempts to establish a concentrically ringed citadel. Each day, the king's laborers would construct a portion of the citadel only to have their work undone by spirits of the land exacting vengeance on behalf of their dethroned monarch. Leading these local spirits was a thousand-year-old white chicken. Eventually, a golden turtle appeared and subdued the white chicken, thereby allowing King An Dương to appropriate the chicken spirit into himself. In some legends King An Dương is even portrayed as a golden chicken (Taylor 1983, 18–22).

According to historian Keith Taylor, these legendary animal exchanges reflect shifting political fortunes in early Vietnam. The underlying theme of the tale is a test of strength between the white chicken, an indigenous Vietnamese symbol of great antiquity, and the golden turtle, a symbol of the Chinese god of war. In Taylor's reading, the chicken occupies a symbolic role in the Vietnamese people's historic efforts to cope with intrusive political leadership.

Taking Taylor's insights further, I want to suggest that poultry, and chickens in particular, are not just symbols of political change and maneuvering. Throughout Vietnamese history, chickens—as living, breathing, corporeal beings—have been important social and political players in Vietnamese people's everyday negotiations of political rule.

Poultry has a long history in Vietnam.[1] Biologists suggest that the chicken was first domesticated from a wild red jungle fowl, *Gallus gallus*, found in South and Southeast Asia, and some archaeological evidence indicates that poultry production began in Vietnam's northern mountain regions around 3,500 years ago (Duc and Long 2008). Traditional "backyard," or "scavenging" production has been the most prevalent chicken rearing system in the country, in which anywhere from a handful to a few dozen birds roam freely in farmers' backyards and gardens, munching on grasses, insects, and seeds. Scavenging birds tend to be *gà ta*, or native, indigenous breeds. In Vietnamese, the pronoun *ta* can refer to I, we, us, my, or our. Added on to the word for chicken, *gà*, *ta* designates something like, "our chicken." This designation is important because it points to the bird's native roots in Vietnam, and because it indicates a sense of ownership over, and community with, the animal. In Vietnam, claims over land and its products, including livestock, are often built on notions of origins and community, and have been critical organizing principles for state agricultural policies as well as citizens' responses to them.

Vietnamese farmers inherit a tradition of using poultry to push back against the effects of exploitative political regimes. Food insecurity has been a mainstay for subjects of both local and foreign rulers in Vietnam, who have variously enacted repressive taxation schemes, abusive labor arrangements, and policies of resource extraction and land dispossession (Goscha 2016).[2] During the Second World War, for instance, the Japanese military invaded Vietnam, then under colonial French control (1887–1945). At the time, typhoons, drought, and flooding coupled with American bombing campaigns to cut off food supplies across the country. French and Japanese occupiers began to use rice and maize to feed troops and fuel power stations. A devastating famine ensued, one that eventually killed upwards of millions of people. A popular fable from the period tells of a young boy and his mother who lived amid these privations. Facing starvation, mother and son dream up plans to build a chicken coop, and the mother promises the boy that soon they will have a large, productive flock and plenty to eat. A message of perseverance and hope in times of hardship and political unrest, this fable points to chicken production as a means of self-sufficiency and a brighter future.

Japan's withdrawal from Southeast Asia and the end of WWII put Vietnamese nationalists (Việt Minh) in a position to wage a war for independence. The First Indochina War resulted in the removal of the French

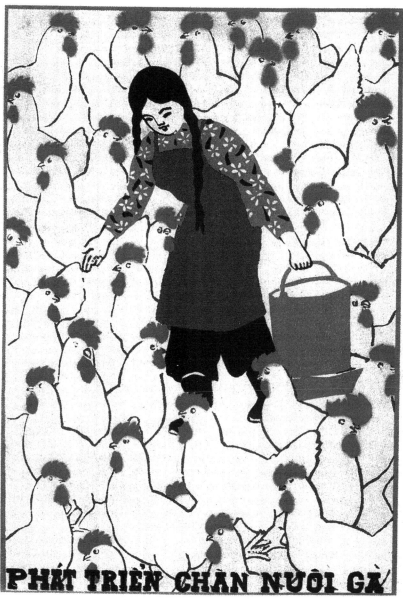

FIG. 1. "Develop chicken production." Propaganda poster promoting rationalized livestock production. Reprinted poster owned and reproduced by author.

colonial government in 1954, and leaders of the newly independent North Vietnam were quick to reclaim plantations owned by colonial landholders and local elites. Under the auspices of putting land back into the hands of the people, North Vietnamese leaders adopted Marxist-Leninist tenets which stated that land should be publicly owned, exploited by cooperatives, and subject to centralized state planning. Though couched in rhetoric of emancipation and reclamation, postcolonial policies put the government in a position to control how agricultural land could be used and how its products could be distributed. Notably, the state turned to livestock, and poultry, as a means to promote these new productive relations. Propaganda posters circulating from the post-WWII period through to the revolutionary and socialist eras included images of industrious farmers raising plump, healthy chickens. Such images accompanied exhortations to develop chicken farming as a way of rebuilding the country, maintaining happy families and villages, and protecting national security.

State policies to collectivize agriculture and seize ownership over land, agricultural goods, and markets further intensified in the period following the Second Indochina War and the reunification of North and South Vietnam under Communist rule in 1975. One particularly impactful policy was the establishment of a subsidy system (*bao cấp*) (1976–86), in which the central government collectivized farms, took control over agricultural products, and distributed food and other goods to citizens in exchange for stamps. Today, the subsidy system is commonly understood to be a spectacular governmental failure, and rural dwellers in particular recall the period as a time of deprivation and vulnerability.

Throughout my stay in Placid Pond village, Thủy and Trí's relatives and neighbors frequently stopped by the house to sit and chat. Among them were Trí's twin nieces. Like most children in the village, Phương and Phúc were slight, their short frames covered by little more than skin darkened by the aggressive sun. Large, protuberant eyes dominated the girls' faces and their mouths were set in protracted grins. I guessed they were about six years old. During one of their visits, however, Thủy informed me that they had just turned fifteen, the same age as her own daughter, Qui. She explained:

> These girls here, you see, their mother grew up during the subsidy period. She was just seventeen or eighteen when she got pregnant and she was already really small, just like Trí. She never had enough to eat growing up. None of us did. Of course we didn't have medical services back then. [Pointing to the nascent bump on her belly] For this baby I go to Bắc Giang city for ultrasounds and supplies, but at that time we didn't do anything different from usual. So Linh [Phương and Phúc's mother] just kept working the rice paddy.

And when she went to deliver we discovered there were two of them. Two little girls! They were so small. Stunted. Linh wasn't eating enough for one, and here there were two. Pitiful! Now look at them, they're half the size they should be. And they're slow.

As was his habit, Trí elaborated on Thủy's comments, "Yeah, Phương and Phúc are small, but they're not that much smaller than Qui. [Sticking up his pinky finger] All the kids their age are just little things (*bé tí*). There's enough to eat now, but when you come out small, you never grow big." Phương and Phúc's diminutive bodies were visual reminders of a period in Placid Pond when food was a constant preoccupation, when bellies cried out for nourishment in spite of farmers' backbreaking labor. Trí's father, Ông Đức, summarized the period this way, "It didn't matter what we produced, there was never enough." Memories of *bao cấp* and its aftereffects now serve as cautionary tales about the negative effects of overreaching government policies.

Placid Pond residents shared many stories about their struggles to exercise a modicum of control over production in the postwar period. Notably, poultry farming became a key means of making do in an increasingly restrictive economy. Some villagers described hiding homegrown chickens from the leaders of farm collectives, and stealing away to slaughter the birds in secret. Other villagers were more enterprising, and Ông Đức prides himself on being the first person in Placid Pond to start a chicken hatchery at the tail end of the subsidy period. Working from his home, he drew on relatives and friends to establish a village-wide trade in eggs and chicks, which he used to supplement state provisions. While Ông Đức oversaw the hatching and incubation process, his wife went door-to-door to exchange eggs and newborn chicks for other goods, a practice she continues to this day. Production grew, and during my stay in Placid Pond Ông Đức owned the largest hatchery in the village.

Ông Đức's hatchery has endured from *bao cấp* through to *đổi mới* economic renovation and now the contemporary Livestock Revolution, but its meaning and value has shifted over time. Since the late 1980s, Vietnam's socialist-led market transition has transformed the contours of rural poultry rearing in the country. Although changing consumption patterns have broadened the scope and intensity of livestock production, the rural economy has faltered under processes of agricultural liberalization and global market integration. Reliance on foreign trade has put agricultural producers in a vulnerable position vis-à-vis international price fluctuations and led to pronounced indebtedness, unemployment, and social inequality (Dollar 2002). What's more, while farmers struggle to produce for an unpredictable and demanding market, their employment opportunities are dwindling in light of state policies that prioritize industrialization and urbanization (Harms 2011; Nguyen and Thomas 2004; Nguyen 2004; Taylor 2007). Small-scale agriculture's share of economic output has continually shrunk over the last four decades, fostering rural unemployment and provoking mass internal and external migrations (Dang 1999; Small 2012; Harms 2011).

These economic policies have had ambivalent effects in Placid Pond. The village forms part of Bắc Giang province, which was repartitioned in 1997 by a rezoning plan that split Ha Bắc province into Bắc Giang, a largely rural area with a few districts attracting foreign manufacturing centers, and Bắc Ninh, a peri-urban region with more developed markets and direct commercial networks with Hanoi to the south. Residents of Placid Pond complained that the government was neglecting to invest in agricultural production and instead pouring more funds into urbanizing areas like Bắc Ninh. As such, they saw no future in farming. Many of the young people I spoke to in the village expressed distaste at the thought of carrying on their family poultry farm, a sentiment their parents shared. Wealthier families paid for tutorial sessions that prepared their children for entrance exams to Hanoi universities, while poorer parents encouraged their kids to seek work in the nearby Korean-owned cosmetic factory, the textile factories bordering the city of Bắc Ninh, or the service sector in Hanoi. More and more families were also pooling resources to send their relatives abroad, paying thousands of US dollars to agents who promised to find them work as factory laborers or as au pairs in Taiwan, Korea, and Greece.

When I moved into Trí and Thủy's house, Thủy had just returned from Taiwan where she had worked as an au pair. Her younger brother as well as her husband's sister and two sisters-in-law were all working abroad at the time of my fieldwork. Such out-migrations were the norm in Placid Pond. It seemed that work anywhere and of any kind was preferable to farming, an endeavor frequently described as miserable (*khổ*) and full of hardship (*vất vả*). Livestock rearing in particular was so unappealing that parents used it to discipline children. Thủy often complained that her daughter was a lazy student, and warned her that if she failed in her studies she would be stuck planting rice and scooping chicken shit. Inheriting a society where Hồ Chí Minh once said that every household should have a garden, a fishpond, and a pig, the rural dwellers I spoke to with proclaimed, "Nobody wants to raise livestock!" (*Không ai muốn chăn nuôi mà!*)

Yet, despite the odds mounting against rural livestock production, poultry persists, and many rural dwellers have intensified production, even if just as a means to provide a different future for their children. It is no accident that Trí and Thủy invested Thủy's earnings into developing their family egg farm, and were saving to send their daughter as well as their neices and nephews to university. Other villagers, too, returned to Placid Pond after a few months or years working as laborers in the capital city, eager to start their own poultry farms. In particular, those who hoped to marry within the village and those who cared for ailing parents were drawn back to the Placid Pond and to poultry farming. Oftentimes, one spouse would care for livestock while the other worked outside of the village, creating a system in which remittances could be funneled back into poultry production.

Everyday economic decisions like these have altered livestock bodies, ecologies, and economies in Vietnam, creating the conditions for pathogens to surface and thrive. These pathogens, in turn, have opened up new opportunities for state, and now multinational, authorities to intervene yet again in rural livelihoods. As I trace emerging forms of One Health governance in rural livestock economies, I remain cognizant of the fact that Vietnam's farmers and leaders have continually looked to poultry, and continually invested in poultry production as a way to exercise control over lives and livelihoods—especially in the context of shifting political-economic conditions. The stories I share will show how notions of community, family, country, ownership, and shared destinies—which have characterized people-poultry relations since the origin of the Vietnamese nation—continue to animate state livestock policies as well as farmers' responses to them. Poultry remain enduring commodities and companions in endeavors to navigate processes of modernization, urbanization, and industrialization in Vietnam, even amid bird flu threats.

Experimental Entrepreneurs

"[Small commercial flocks] are a feature of urbanizing societies or economies that are beginning to grow. . . . There is a general consensus that stricter biosecurity is needed for these flocks but it needs to be implemented in a way that helps the more entrepreneurial farmers to adopt new measures, using incremental steps rather than sudden changes. . . . If increased productivity could be demonstrated, this could become the incentive to apply biosecurity" (Honhold et al. 2008, 33–35).

This statement comes from a report by the United Nations Food and Agricultural Organization (FAO), which details options for implementing biosecurity procedures to protect human and nonhuman animals from harmful agents. Based on field studies of poultry production in Africa, Europe, and Asia, the report finds that biosecurity entails significant financial investments, and will therefore be most successful if taken up by risk-taking, entrepreneurial producers. What's more, these imagined entrepreneurs are more likely to be motivated by increased productivity than by disease vulnerability, which means that biosecurity proponents should try to show a correlation between pathogen control and poultry output. This short excerpt clearly encapsulates how bird flu programmers align the interests of global public health with those of commercial livestock production. For the FAO, a key champion of One Health, the cultivation of flu-free poultry goes hand in hand with its commercialization.

I begin this story of bird flu governance with an examination of two biosecure farms, the first involving ducks and the second involving chickens. Each of these farms entails experimental modifications to poultry biology and ecologies, which in turn restructure how poultry interact with each other, farmers, and consumers. In what follows, I detail the novel exchanges between people, poultry, and pathogens that surface on biosecure farms, and consider the implications of these exchanges for the different actors involved. I contend that biosecurity experiments mark an emergent mode of health programming, which unites biological and commercial objectives, and envisions a future of livestock farming characterized by outbreak reduction *and* enhanced production. I further argue that by bridging health and commerce, biosecurity experiments mark a shift in how health workers understand and value health subjects. Namely, biosecurity proponents promote fowl more in terms of market viability than biological vulnerability, and they treat farmers more like enterprising entrepreneurs than susceptible smallholders. Among the results of biosecurity experiments, then, are new valuations that determine who will be biologically and economically secure.

Agriculture and environmental specialists began using the term "biosecurity" in the 1990s in response to foot-and-mouth disease outbreaks in the United Kingdom and related fears of bioterror. The term gained force in the wake of the September 11, 2001, attacks in the United States and the subsequent release of anthrax to government and media outlets. Since then, biosecurity has become a highly charged concept spanning the domains of public health, agriculture, and national security. It conjures an image of global bio-communicability, in which danger lurks within and across all kinds of boundaries (Sharp and Chen 2014). Bruce Braun puts it nicely when he says that biosecurity conceives of a human body "embedded in a chaotic and unpredictable molecular world, a body understood in terms of a genetic economy of exchange and circulation, haunted by the specter of newly emerging or still indefinable risks" (Braun 2007, 14).

Biosecurity is all about coping with exchange and circulation. But in the context of livestock economies, biosecurity is less about blocking biological exchanges than it is about promoting "good" biological exchanges (Hinchliffe, Enticott, and Bingham 2008). Livestock is livestock precisely because it is meant to enter into networks of exchange relations and market transactions. It must move. Strategies to securitize livestock pathogens must therefore occur alongside a broader effort to traffic in their carriers (Donaldson 2008; Enticott 2008). This is not an easy task, because risky interspecies exchanges often overlap with economically productive ones. On poultry farms in particular, biosecurity emerges in what Allen and Lavau (2015) call a *relational economy* of disease, in which measures to enhance productivity (such as increasing flock densities or using antibiotics) create an evolving landscape of harmful agents and commercial processes. Put simply, in livestock economies, good economic exchanges can also foster dangerous biological ones.

Because biosecurity intervenes in overlapping and sometimes incompatible health and economic sectors, its efficacy is difficult to define and measure. At the time of my fieldwork (and up until today), it remains unclear if biosecurity measures actually prevent bird flu. The report I opened with states:

> To date, there has been little work completed on the role of improved biosecurity in slowing down the spread of HPAI or on how sustainable biosecurity measures are likely to be. There has been little involvement of those who will have to implement biosecurity to assess which, if any, measures are practical and sustainable, or whether enhanced biosecurity is likely to be adopted. There are few examples of best practices or results of trials. These are all key areas that need to be addressed (Honhold et al. 2008, 10).

Bird flu programmers in Vietnam were concerned about the uncertainty surrounding biosecurity, and in 2009 the FAO and the Vietnamese Department of Animal Health launched a working group to create a list of good practices biosecurity guidelines to try, or experiment with, in affected communities. An FAO advisor told me that the guidelines would address inconsistent information about biosecurity and provide a standard set of practices that could be adapted to farms of different sizes and with different poultry breeds. To get started on the guidelines, the FAO office in Hanoi invited the lead author of the above biosecurity report to convene a workshop to discuss key biosecurity principles and how they might be tested in the Vietnamese context. He arrived in the capital just a few months after publishing the report, and his visit comprised part of a global pilgrimage to introduce his findings to affected nations.

The author, a veterinary specialist, began the workshop by focusing attention on the ever-present pathogenic potential of the "human-animal interface." He stated that anthropogenic changes to animal ecosystems are the primary drivers of pathogen emergence and proliferation. "The disease is mostly spread by the action of man [sic], moving either infected birds or contaminated materials." Biosecurity, he explained, addresses the risky interspecies interface by taking the public health principle of social distancing and applying it across species. This means enclosing uninfected poultry through barriers that limit contact with outside agents; cleaning tools and objects that come into contact with poultry and poultry products; and disinfecting production areas before bringing new flocks onto the farm. Together, these measures restrict pathogen circulation by reducing poultry's proximities to other potentially infectious animals and materials, both human and nonhuman.

Importantly, the measures that the consultant introduced in Hanoi were not meant to be unique to Vietnam, but rather constituted a first step in an ongoing agenda for global livestock securitization. Developed by the FAO in collaboration with the World Organization for Animal Health (OIE), the global biosecurity agenda recommends compartmentalizing infection-free poultry within a standardized transnational governance system, and then zoning those birds into regions far removed from birds whose health status is unknown (World Organization for Animal Health 2015). On this view, biosecurity is both a biological and commercial endeavor, one that limits global trade to epidemiologically circumscribed species varieties or what the OIE calls "disease free" poultry subpopulations.

Experimental Life

Biosecurity is global in scope but locally adaptive; it's a principal intervention for bird flu, but its capacity to stem infection is unclear; and it seeks to bridge health and economic objectives, even though they are often at odds with one another. In all of these ways, biosecurity exemplifies the experimental ethos of bird flu governance. In Vietnam, on-the-farm biosecurity interventions test unproven ways of governing people-poultry-pathogen relations in order to gather information about their feasibility down the road. In doing so, they draw together different actors (vets, public health workers, farmers, and fowl), each with their own unique ways of addressing harmful biological agents. These experiments happen in situ: they modify existing exchanges between people and poultry as a means to investigate future options for securitizing *and* commoditizing life.

Addressing pathogens and productivity in equal measure, biosecurity experiments take a multipronged approach that includes *biologically* designing birds to increase their immunity, and *socially* situating them in new exchange relations with humans. To capture the poultry varieties and the people-poultry relations that surface on biosecure farms, I also take a multipronged approach, and elaborate a distinction between *life forms* and *forms of life*. Anthropologist Stefan Helmreich defines life forms as "embodied bits of vitality called organisms, variously apprehended as ranged into species," and forms of life as "cultural, social, symbolic, and pragmatic ways of thinking and acting that organize human communities" (2009, 6). Put simply, a life form is a living organism and a form of life is a way of living. Though distinct, I suggest that life forms and forms of life mutually constitute each other, and I am interested in how they do so in bird flu experiments; in this case on biosecure farms.

Life forms and forms of life are both ripe for experimentation. Stefan Helmreich and Sophia Roosth show that life form signals possibilities for how life might take shape. Life form conjures dual notions: of a bounded being capable of self-organization and self-regulation; and of an elastic being constantly adjusting to material circumstances (2016, 19, 24). Over time, scientists have imagined myriad ways that life can form in different settings and in response to different catalysts, and there is a long history of fashioning organisms according to evolving views about their capacity to affect, and be affected by, environments (Biesel and Boete 2013; Creager 2001; Davies 2011, 2012, 2013; Kohler 1994; Leonelli and Ankeny 2013; Ankeny et al. 2014; Lezaun and Porter 2015 Nading 2014a, 2014b; Nelson 2013, 2018; Rader 2004).

For anthropologists, sociocultural ideas and practices play a decisive role in the forms that life takes, and many have used *forms of life* to capture this dynamic. First developed by Ludwig Wittgenstein, a form of life is a social agreement or convention that guides how individuals perceive and respond to the worlds around them. Veena Das defines a form of life as a complicated agreement—an entanglement of rules, customs, habits, examples, and practices that defines a person's belonging in a culture as well as their ability to express themselves in that culture (1998, 176). Importantly, forms of life guide thought and action, but they are not entirely pre-determined or determining. "One might say that life has a pulsating, dynamic quality and that the question of what it is to have agreement in a form of life is not a matter settled once and for all, but has to be secured by the work done every day" (Cavell, in Das 2016, 170). Forms of life, in other words, are flexible, and this is particularly true in times of uncertainty. Michael Fischer uses *emergent forms of life* to describe everyday renegotiations that occur in the face of new problems. Using pandemics as one example, he suggests that such problems prompt affected communities to establish new relations of production and consumption and adopt new modes of thinking and feeling (Fischer 2005, 55; see also Zhan 2005). This work is messy. In emergent forms of life, different voices intersect and collide, objects and facts compete for authority, and new rules of play come into being.

Just like life forms, forms of life point to possibilities and problem solving; and just like life forms, they are open to tinkering and transformation. Experimentation. I want to bring these concepts together to explore how new life forms come into being *alongside* new forms of life on experimental, biosecure farms. This means pushing forms of life past the human communities they're most often associated with (Hartigan 2015), and considering the unsettled agreements that surface among humans and nonhumans facing pandemic flu together.[1] It also means asking how biosecure chickens and ducks habituate to poultry producing arrangements, while at the same time expressing capacious vitalities (Helmreich and Roosth 2016, 21) that are capable of transforming those arrangements along the way.

Model Ducks

I begin with the model ducks I encountered on biosecure farms in Đồng Tháp province in the Mekong Delta. These ducks comprised part of an integrated fish-duck farm, which sought to convert free-range duck production into an enclosed and more secure farming system. The traditional mode of duck production in the Mekong Delta consists of ducks moving from rice paddy to rice paddy, feeding on snails, insects, and crabs at various stages of rice maturation. As they do so, they till the fields and excrete vital nutrients that help the rice grow. Though they save money and labor, the introduction of mechanized cultivation and faster growing, pest-resistant rice varieties has put free-range ducks' long-term survival into question. As early as the 1970s, state agricultural experts in Vietnam began investigating ways to redirect the productive potential of free-range ducks, and engaged in research and experiments to integrate duck and fish production. This work was suspended during the Second Indochina War, but has gained more attention in the last few decades and is now a key focus of bird flu programs promoted by the state in collaboration with the FAO and other partners.

Though there are local variations, the basic structure of these farms includes a fully enclosed duck coop built at a predefined distance from a bordered pond containing various kinds of fish. The ducks spend the night in the coops, but during daylight hours they are let into the pond where they scavenge for plankton and any other edibles assembling around the ducks. Just as they would in rice paddies, biosecure ducks excrete manure that enriches pond water and provides nutrients to fish. Farmers provide the ducks with a daily ration of certified commercial feed, but the idea is that grazing ducks require less sustenance and thereby allow farmers to save money. Model ducks don't just promise to cut costs; they are also supposed to increase income. This is because their avian labor forms the foundation for producing fish, a secondary livestock product that is often more lucrative than ducks.

It's easy to see how this system would attract biosecurity proponents keen to reach entrepreneurial farmers. Applying biosecurity principles to integrated fish-duck farms entails creating physical barriers and effecting social distancing measures to prevent the introduction and circulation of harmful agents. Biosecure fish-duck farms use space as well as netting, concrete, and other materials to protect duck coops and fish ponds from unwanted contact with outside agents. They also use as standardized feeding, health care, and cleaning practices that limit the interactions that ducks can have with farmers, fish, and each other.

In principle, these biosecurity measures seem straightforward. But these are real world experiments that gain their own life on the ground. A few months after I began my fieldwork in Đồng Tháp, the provincial veterinarian responsible for helping me carry out my research, Hạnh, invited me to join her on a visit to a few model duck farms. The farms were being piloted by a multinational NGO based in Ho Chi Minh City in collaboration with Đồng Tháp's provincial and district-level veterinary departments. Hạnh explained that each month the NGO sent over representatives to check in on the progress of the farms and that she was responsible for escorting the visitors to the sites. She seemed miffed that she would have to spend all day with the representatives, which surprised me because Hạnh usually tackled her daily responsibilities with alacrity.

We began the day in a briefing session at the Provincial People's Committee Office, where I met Hiển, Mỹ, and Thaí. Hiển and Mỹ had come from the multinational NGO's headquarters in Ho Chi Minh City. Hiển was the project manager for the farm models and Mỹ was working in a supportive role. Both had training in the social sciences and international development. It was their third time in the province. Thái was a state-employed veterinarian in the district where the models were being piloted. He was the one responsible for making sure that the daily operations of the farms were up to spec. As the group began going over the schedule for the site visits, Thái shared some bad news. He informed us that of the eleven households initially participating in the biosecure-farming program, seven had pulled out. The problem, he explained, was that the variety of duck introduced on the biosecure farms was not suitable for this environment. Unlike the hybrid duck common to the area, apparently this variety struggled to survive in the southern climate and failed to fetch the market price promised by the NGO.

"People here don't want to invest in biosecurity because the profit isn't assured."

"Yeah," Hạnh added, "Just because the model worked in An Giang [province] doesn't mean it will here. Plus, the contract for this program is too long. Even we [vets] don't read all the guidelines. How can we expect the farmers to?"

Hiển shot back, "You need to interpret it for them. . . . You have to educate them! And tell them that only those with resources should farm poultry. Ultimately this is a project to *prevent bird flu, not to promote economics.*"

Hiển's attempt to mark a distinction between bird flu prevention and

commercial gain seemed ironic to me. My observations of other bird flu interventions as well as biosecurity strategizing sessions in Hanoi had all revealed a concerted effort on behalf of bird flu programmers to align virus
control with increased productivity and profit. Indeed, all of the bird flu programs I observed conceived of farmers as rational economic actors pursuing
higher profits and better livelihoods. But as I was to learn on this day, economic and health interests sometimes failed to link up in practice.

As the briefing went on, I learned that the model ducks were disease-free
poultry populations raised on farms that had taken the FAO's biosecurity
principles and adapted them to the Mekong Delta ecology. Hiền showed me
an image of the principles in action. It depicted the farm's key features: a
coop, yard, and pond. The pond was separated from the coop by at least six
meters in order to deter waterborne microbial transfer (ideally any pathogen
will perish in the time it takes to cover the distance). Three walls, a fence,
and a roof enclosed the coop, the feeding troughs near the pond were also
contained, and each farm component was separated from the other through
a strategic placement of fences. Further, the entire system was distanced from
the household, roads, and neighbors that were labeled, but too far away to
appear in the picture. Social distancing materialized in this idealized image as
a series of species separations, with spatial and structural barriers preventing
poultry from coming into contact with other animals (including humans)
outside of the biosecure space.

The farms I visited with Hạnh were laid out in a similar fashion. The duck
flocks, a hundred or two hundred in number, waded at the edge of small,
shallow ponds about ten meters square, dug about twenty meters from the
household. Nylon fencing surrounded their enclosures, reaching up a few
feet all around and down a few feet to the bottom of the ponds. The pond
edges nearest the coops were cemented like a swimming pool and acted as a
staging area where ducks could enter the water from their coops. The coops
themselves were enclosed with aluminum roofs that opened on one end to
the staging areas. The ponds were large enough for the ducks to kick their
feet several times before wading into one another, though the animals I saw
at each farm were either in their coops or clustered together at the edge of the
ponds away from the open water. I was told that twice a day farmers scattered
pre-measured commercial feed around the body of water for the ducks to
feed on. At night, the birds slept in their coops.

Each week the ducks and their farmers received an unannounced visit
from Thái (and any other veterinary agents, traveling NGO workers, or anthropologists who happened to come along). Thái's job was to weigh a model
duck to check its growth rate against the commercial brand standard, as well

as fill out a checklist that documented whether the ducks' food and antibiotic administration were on schedule. He also took blood samples to test for H5N1. Finally, Thái asked the farmer a series of predetermined questions about the feeding habits of the animals and their reaction to various environmental factors. If the NGO workers were around, they might pose a few more questions for Thái to ask, focusing on any troubles the farmers had run into with regard to farm upkeep. If present, the NGO workers would round out the visit by snapping shots to take back to headquarters for the production of glossy pamphlets and monitoring and evaluation reports for their funders. This was Mỹ's task, and she enjoyed toting the large camera around, capturing images of the fowl and her friends.

At one of the farms, the farmer fed the flock to demonstrate their appetite levels and eating habits. The birds had been resting under their canopied coop but when he opened it up to the staging area, or "play yard" (sân chơi), they emerged en masse into the open area. At first they didn't seem to be moving much. It was crowded in the play yard, almost brimming with birds. It looked as if they were adjusting to the light of the sunshine. The farmer walked through the flock waving his arms slowly. The ducks took the cue and moved as if shepherded toward the edge of the pond. Here, instead of the gradual slope from walking path to rice paddy that free-range ducks enjoy, the birds eased themselves into the water via a cemented incline that connected the play yard to the pond. I noted that while free-range paddy ducks would often stay at the water's edge where lily pads and other loose grasses collected, snacking on snails and insects hidden in the foliage, here there was no greenery to attract the ducks' attention and of course no rice grasses for them to weave in and out of. Those ducks positioned closest to the water walked down slowly, and then sort of floated in small groups just about a foot or so from the edge. They did not immediately dunk their heads in search of food or break off into smaller groups to graze. Rather, they looked around at each other and the rest of the flock. To me they seemed exposed.

When the farmer threw in the feed, though, the activity began. The ducks kicked their webbed feet to get at the pellets ahead of the others. The food flew in an arc formation from the farmer's hand so that it sailed over the expanse of the pond. While the ducks initially swam toward the farmer, as the pellets splashed both in front of and behind them, they began to stay somewhat stationary, moving in concentric circles to get at the pellets in their vicinity. The fish, too, began popping their heads up to the surface, and the water seemed to bubble up around the ducks as the fish went for the feed. The ducks, in turn, kicked a bit harder to get at the pellets and, I guessed, to free up some space between them and the gulping fish. When the feed was exhausted, the fish moved back down into the water. The ducks kicked around a bit more, and then let themselves fall still. Pairs of two or three would float alongside one another, but I couldn't tell if this was intentional or the outcome of the water's current moving them in unison. I was told that as the ducks digested and defecated, they would provide more nutrients for the hungry fish. I asked Hạnh how the birds seemed to her and she said their weight looked normal for their age, and that their appetites were satisfactory. There were not any particularly sickly or lethargic-looking birds either. She said nothing about their social activity or mood.

During the site visits farmers also dutifully presented their "Monitoring the Flock" journals to veterinary staff, showing how carefully they had recorded their ducks' vital statistics. Yet, even as they presented evidence of "good farm management" to veterinarians and NGO workers, they did not seem entirely on board with the project. Some asked: Why? Why are we feeding Carhill feed? Why are we giving antibiotics? Why can't the ducks graze in the yard or in the nearby rice paddies? Why are you taking all this information when it doesn't affect the sale price? These questions were germane, because in many ways the biosecure duck's lifestyle was diametrically opposed to the forms of life common to the Mekong Delta. In the first instance, duck enclosures were inconsistent with a duck-rice growing economy that depends upon the free and expansive *movements* of poultry. Many duck farmers in this and other southern provinces practiced a form of cultivation wherein farmers and flocks walk, ride, or wade to neighboring rice paddies to feed. In fact, some farmers saw the enclosure of birds as a health hazard. *Chật*, cramped, was a term they frequently used to describe the walled coops and fenced-in canopies characteristic of model farms. In one of my other visits to a model farm, a farmer pulled me aside, pointed to a biosecure coop, and asked, "How can you tell if the birds are sick when they're all crammed together inside like that? They could die and we wouldn't even notice!"

In the second instance, the model ducks inhabiting these enclosures were a foreign, commercial variety that is more difficult and expensive to procure than the hybrids common to southern poultry economies. Producing the model life form according to biosecure, commercial standards required restructuring farm space (erecting enclosures and adding ponds if needed), administering commercial brand medical and alimentary inputs, and submitting to the watchful eyes of state vets and non-state flu strategists. Farmers seemed particularly wary of biosecure feeding strategies since commercial feed was not only expensive, but also often associated with hazardous chemicals. When concentrated in small ponds, these chemicals were considered even more dangerous.

As I watched the farmer sprinkling Carhill feed into the water, I was reminded of a fable that Thủy had shared with me when I lived in Placid Pond. It told of the trials of a Vietnamese woman who marries into a rich foreign family. When the young bride relocates to her in-laws' house, she finds herself surrounded by a grove of magnificent custard apple, or soursop, trees, whose gargantuan fruit hang low and heavy over a crystal-clear pond. The bride is told that when the custard apples fall from the tree into the pond, the fruit becomes imbued with a special preservative that allows the family to sell the fruit in markets far and wide. One day the young woman decides to sample a floating delicacy. But when she reaches into the pond her skin begins to burn and bubble, peeling from her arm in sheets and disintegrating into what she only then realizes is a pool of toxic chemicals. When Thủy related the fable to me, she did so as a cautionary tale about foreign foodstuffs and their purveyors. I didn't ask the southern farmers what they thought about the story, but I felt its message went some way in explaining their reluctance to employ unfamiliar feeding regimes.

The confluence of the breed, structural inputs, and biometrics in this experiment indicated a standard of productivity and security that distinguished the model duck as an infection-free investment. But this biosecure life form came alongside a form of life that weaved prophylactics and profit in ways that some viewed as a threat. Hạnh complained that the farmers didn't care about how much the bird is supposed to weigh at weeks one, two, and three, that they just wanted to know the reasons for biosecurity and how all of these measures would help them turn a profit. Hạnh was right to point out that the farmers, vets, and NGO workers had different expectations about the experiment's results. They didn't agree. Farmers wanted to know when the biosecure inputs would fetch a higher price for their fowl. Hiền and Mỹ, on the other hand, were looking for data to bring back to the NGO (and its funder) that would shed light on the viability of this experimental type of duck production. Biometric data, photographs, and farmers' comments on their experiences comprised the results of the biosecurity experiment and the empirical basis for funder decisions about whether to implement the experiment elsewhere, modify it, or scrap it in favor of another one.

Such an outward-looking experimental agenda was a point of contention between NGO workers and veterinarians. Hiền and Mỹ were in the province in order to evaluate whether there were any "local obstacles" that they could address when introducing the model ducks elsewhere. When Hạnh and Thái suggested that the main obstacle was lack of investment, and asked for 26 billion Vietnamese Đông from the NGO in order take over long-term management of the project, Hiền said that it was the responsibility of the

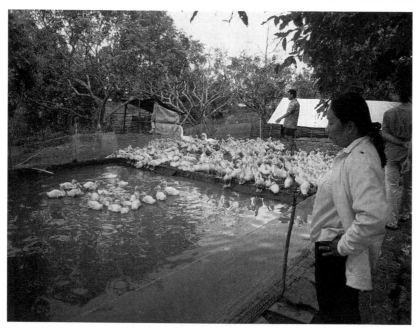

FIG. 2. Hạnh inspects a model duck farm in Đồng Tháp Province. The ducks have been let out of their enclosure and are entering the artificial pond to feed. Photo by author.

province to continue financing the farms. Unbeknownst to Hạnh and Thái, the NGO was not actually concerned with overcoming the obstacles *in Đồng Tháp*; they merely wanted to document them as experimental outcomes, or "lessons learned." The local only mattered insofar as it could be made into a controlled variable for future experiments.

Naturally Vietnam Chickens

Yet there are other life forms and forms of life at play in biosecurity experiments, those that call more on local tradition and taste. In 2009, a major US development agency launched a avian flu initiative comprised in part by a project to bring hygienic, biosecure poultry farming practices in line with "traditional" farming methods. Out of this initiative came a new brand of Naturally Vietnam chicken, the "first premium quality label for traceable food made in Vietnam." Like the model ducks in Đồng Tháp, Naturally Vietnam chickens drew on and modified free-ranging poultry-rearing practices. Chicken production in Vietnam has historically been characterized by "backyard" or "scavenging" farming systems, in which families produce a small flock of birds for household consumption. These birds graze for insects and other edibles in backyards, often retiring to a makeshift chicken coop to sleep and lay eggs. A defining feature of backyard chickens is that they are *gà ta*, or native varieties (or else native-commercial hybrids). *Gà ta* are thought to be particularly well-suited to scavenging; they are slimmer, taller, slower grow-ing, and more agile than top-heavy, fast-to-fatten commercial birds. Such a biological makeup complements a free-ranging form of life to make backyard birds appear healthier and tastier to consumers.

The donor and its partners recognized the consumer preferences and therefore market potential for traditional chicken, and devised an experi-ment that aimed to both securitize and commoditize Vietnam's beloved backyard bird. Developed by two veterinarians living in Hanoi, a European expatriate and his Vietnamese wife, Naturally Vietnam chickens were dis-tinguished by several characteristics that combine biological security with consumer preference. These chickens were raised in free-range production systems where they had daily access to expansive, but enclosed, outdoor gar-dens. These were not really backyards, but rather larger spaces set at some distance from households. Here, the birds ate plants and insects, but they were also given commercial feed with minimal genetic modifications. And unlike traditional backyard birds who require minimal upkeep, these chick-ens underwent weekly tests for H5N1 exposure as well as antibiotic residue. They were also slaughtered away from the household, in facilities adhering to the newest European Union hygiene standards.

Like all biosecure livestock forms, Naturally Vietnam chickens were eval-uated according to their biological and commercial value. But in addition to these quantifiable bio-commercial properties, Naturally Vietnam chick-ens also embodied qualitative indices of tradition and taste. In a press re-lease circulated to HPAI strategists, a farmer reflects: "Raising chickens was not new to us. But this is the first time we have learned not only how to produce healthy free-range chickens but also to slaughter them according to principles of good hygiene and food safety assurance." Another press re-lease stated, "The Naturally Vietnam approach allows Vietnamese farmers to produce safe and tasty meat and eggs while preserving the environment and their incomes." Health security manifested here in principled and profit-able exchanges between people and poultry. And while they resulted in novel life forms (the trademarked Naturally Vietnam brand), these exchanges also drew on well-established ways of living with poultry in Vietnam.

Naturally Vietnam chickens were discursively situated in economies where taste and tradition overlapped with health and productivity as markers of value. A marketing leaflet related the story of Mr. Sang, who drew on his traditional production expertise to breed a "unique chicken that combined

slow growth, delicious meat, high production capacity and good uniformity."
Unlike model ducks, these life forms are given time and room to grow. This
is a mark of distinction, one that separated Naturally Vietnam chickens from
hyper-productive, fast-growing commercial varieties being introduced on
model duck and other farms all over Vietnam. Further, unlike model ducks,
Naturally Vietnam fowl enjoyed a variety of feed sources that promoted their
health and welfare. A primary marketing angle of the Naturally Vietnam
brand was the fact that the chickens' diet largely consisted of plant and insect
sources augmented by commercial feed with minimal genetic enhancements
and antibiotic additions (the types of additives that concerned model duck
farmers). What was entrepreneurial about biosecure chickens, then, was not
so much their built-in productivity, but rather their consumer appeal.

I was not able to visit any Naturally Vietnam chicken farms, in part because of my travel schedule, but also in part because developers were trying to
discourage unnecessary contact between poultry and people. In a biosecurity
workshop in Hanoi, the brand's co-creator warned audiences that bringing
donor representatives, NGO workers, and other stakeholders onto farms create opportunities for microbial transfer, either by carrying pathogens onto
farms, or carrying them away to new sites. "Too many times I have seen my
colleagues walk into slaughterhouses and farms without booties and leave
without washing shoes or hands. If we're really serious about controlling
HPAI, we need to limit contact."

Although I did not see the birds for myself, I was able to view some of the
videos that Naturally Vietnam staff had taken of the farms. What struck me
first was the size of the free-ranging space. The farms in the videos had at least
seventy square meters of space for a few scores of chickens to graze in (far
larger than any of the farms I saw in Placid Pond). Enclosed by chicken wire
fencing, the spaces were covered in lush grasses and shady tree areas. The
chickens huddled together in small groups under the shade, looking at each
other and in the grasses for food, plucking here and there for seeds and bugs.
The birds circled around one another, exacting at least a few inches of space
between their bodies, or else nudging up against each other to reach for the
piles of feed the farmer had just thrown their way. There were other spaces,
too, with canopied structures and water troughs hanging from above. This is
where the birds seemed to spend most of their time, moving in and out from
beneath the canopy to the shaded tree-lined area adjacent to it. The viewer
could hear the breeze blowing and see the leaves and grasses rustling.

I was also struck by the dissimilarity between the Naturally Vietnam farms
and the chicken farms belonging to Thủy and Trí in Placid Pond. Thủy and
Trí kept their birds in their backyard and in the backyard of close relatives.

But their chickens were not freewheeling scavengers. Their chickens resided in much smaller enclosures covered by corrugated metal and walled on three sides by brick. The enclosures were perpetually shaded, but dark, and the only breeze was provided by a single fan. The birds jostled for space and kicked at each other, causing feathers and feces to fly up and out into the air, getting picked up and recirculated by the fan. Thủy and Trí's hens also seemed to move en masse. When Thủy or I would throw feed their way, they ran toward it in unison, moving first in a beeline at one angle, pecking at the feed, and then jettisoning off in a beeline at a different angle to the next batch of feed, and on and on. The chickens I observed on fully commercialized chickens farms also had their own forms of socializing and moving through space. They would gather around the feed troughs hanging at patterned distances from one another, spacing themselves out but staying at one trough rather than moving around to feed from different sources. When the troughs were emptied, the birds moved just about a foot away and plopped down on their haunches; they did not seem to pair off or form any kind of grouping that I could observe, either when eating or when moving around their enclosure. In fact, they seemed rather antagonistic. In Placid Pond and in larger commercial farms, birds would peck and kick at each other as they jostled for food, so much so that Trí and Thủy used a sautering iron to dull the tips of their beaks to avoid injury. I learned that this was a common technique for managing chicken sociality on densely populated farms.

Naturally Vietnam chickens, on the other hand, seemed to have more opportunities to carve out their own social and ecological arrangements. Though uniform in breed, the birds distinguished themselves in their interactions with each other, farmers, and the landscape. Some birds in the video would move in twos to graze, distancing themselves for a time from the flock in order to feed; others would back themselves into outward facing circles in the corners of the canopied areas; still others seemed to roam around on their own, pecking at the feet of their comrades and eliciting clucks in response. I noted that, unlike the chickens in Placid Pond, these birds had not had their beak tips shunted. I guessed that these bodily alerations were unnecessary, because Naturally Vietnam chickens had larger spaces around which to create more cohesive and agreeable social arrangements. The birds also seemed more active. An ad circular stated that the chickens "fully express their natural behavior in contact with the ground and the plants in the open air." While I am not interested in measuring these chickens' naturalness against commercial breeds, I did notice clear differences in *and an attention to* their forms of life—their social behaviors, bodily movements, and ecological habituations.

Although the lifestyle activities and alimentary inputs associated with free-ranging have not been quantifiably shown to reduce H5N1 infection rates, in interviews Naturally Vietnam promoters suggested that these production techniques kept toxins writ large from entering poultry and human bodies alike. The developer of Naturally Vietnam chickens told me that in addition to avian flu, one of the main health risks from Vietnamese chickens was the presence of antibiotics from medicated food sources, and as such Naturally Vietnam chickens ate antibiotic-free commercial feed, and underwent weekly tests for antibiotic residues. Here, then, production practices linked health security to a quantifiable measure of "naturalness." Free-ranging, slow-growing, and unmedicated, Naturally Vietnam chickens took form in highly conscripted, biosecure systems where their productivity rates and health status emerged in conjunction with other indicators of value, including their enrollment in traditional forms of poultry keeping, and, of course, their tastiness.

Importantly, the cultivation processes that engendered the Naturally Vietnam chicken precluded its adoption in global livestock markets. The brand's developer told me that even though Vietnamese consumers overwhelmingly prefer backyard chicken, at the time there was a very small domestic market for biosecure backyard varieties. This was because consumer demand for certifiably safe meat remained nascent in Vietnam. "The average chicken consumer is motivated by price, appearance, and relationships with vendors." He added, "You know, we really haven't mentioned H5N1 in the last two years." In this local context, at least for the majority of consumers, quantifiable demonstrations of disease resistance lost force as markers of value. And so although Naturally Vietnam chickens were certifiably H5N1 free, in order to expand their market base developers drew on other indicators of value: yellow skin, firm thighs, and chewy meat. They further linked these attributes to free-range, traditional production methods. As a press release had it, this lifestyle "gives more flavor and texture to the meat, . . . [while] industrial chicken meat [is] without flavor and too tender."

Questions of what constitutes nature and artifice aside, this branding practice linked the biological immunity of chickens, farmers, and consumers together in experimental forms of life animated by ideals about how people and poultry should live with each other in Vietnam. A very different logic thus drove this biosecurity experiment: it tested a site-specific mode of security firmly situated in domestic poultry markets with unique multispecies exchange relationships. The life form created under the Naturally Vietnam brand was not enrolled in a program of species competition in which the strongest, most productive, and profitable varieties survive.

Rather, it emerged in a regime of species preservation that sought to uphold locally specific farming traditions and locally specific life forms.

But how Vietnamese were these chickens? Naturally Vietnam varieties were actually not *gà ta*, the highly valued native variety first domesticated in and unique to Asia. In fact, Naturally Vietnam's developer contended that in a poultry economy where interbreeding is common and unregulated, native *gà ta* no longer exist: there is no pure genetic line of local chicken in Vietnam. Instead, the Naturally Vietnam brand is a *rouge*, RedBro broiler chicken, a heritage breed from France distributed internationally by corporate breeders like Hubbard. Like *gà ta*, the breed is known for its slow growth and tastiness. And yet, Vietnamese consumers were not sold on RedBro. The brand's developer told me that even though so-called local breeds perform terribly vis-à-vis *rouge* breed, "there is still quite a loyalty to so-called *gà ta*, so we're trying some things to promote the *rouge* chicken." While the brand's marketing materials suggested that this variety was thriving in Vietnam's free-range farming milieus, I was reminded of the unfortunate fate of the foreign duck variety introduced on Đồng Tháp's biosecure farms, which farmers complained struggled both in local climates and markets. This is not to suggest that the RedBro variety was doomed to fail in Vietnam, but it is to point out that many producers and consumers associated tradition with local breeds. Many also suggested that while *gà ta* thrive on rice grasses and backyard insects, such food sources were not suitable for foreign varieties that require expensive feed to survive.[2] For all its emphasis on place, the Naturally Vietnam chicken raised questions about what life forms and associated forms of life belonged in Vietnam's multispecies communities.

Value-Added Poultry and the Entrepreneurial Ethos

Model ducks and Naturally Vietnam varieties are both examples of how zoonotic biosecurity generated new kinds of experimental life forms. Having fallen under the purview of One Health governance, poultry was undergoing significant biophysical transformations in the name of security and productivity. Alongside these novel life forms came experimental forms of life, or ways of living with other species in a pandemic age. The vital properties of biosecure ducks and chickens were enacted and sustained by humans and in particular social arrangements, habits, and practices that sought to realize the animals' commercial potential while simultaneously stemming infection.

I want to suggest that these experimental forms of life imagined novel kinds of health subjects. Global public health has recently been understood as a process that creates patron-client relationships: health workers talk about being in contractual relationships with "client" populations, in which each party brings particular obligations and expectations to the table. Susan Reynolds Whyte and colleagues call this "therapeutic clientship," and show how global health resources get distributed through relationships of obligation and expectation between health workers and vulnerable populations (2013, 151). In therapeutic clientship, health is not a right available to all; rather, it is only open to those individuals who can successfully negotiate a moral economy of patronage.

The biosecurity experiments described here also established contractual relationships between health workers and vulnerable populations, but these relationships were commercial in nature. It is no accident that Đồng Tháp's biosecure duck farmers signed physical contracts with NGO workers that held them and their ducks to particular production standards. Certainly these relationships were imbued with morally inflected expectations and obligations. But the stakes were different. Biosecure farmers did not just make themselves available to health services, but they also engaged in and resisted entrepreneurial forms of life that included new exchange relationships with health workers, commercial actors, consumers, and poultry. Poultry also engaged in these entrepreneurial forms of life; they habituated, and learned to make place in new ecologies and with new human and nonhuman companions. Farmers and fowl, then, were not just the recipients of health interventions; they actively shaped the fields of experimentation. But farmers and fowl also shouldered the risks of experimentation: farmers could lose clients or income, and fowl could lose freedom of movement, opportunities to grow, and their lives. In these experiments, neither health nor profits were available to all, but rather only to those who could successfully turn a profit. Put another way, biosecurity experiments economized life in such a way that those who deserved to live as livestock farmers were those who could properly commoditize ducks and chickens: those who could successfully bring commercial forms to life. An individual's value, their livelihood, and their health, were all tied to the value of their poultry product.

Contract duck farmers in Đồng Tháp have felt the costs more than the benefits of the biosecure farm model. Model ducks were a risky undertaking. They required considerable resources to both procure and produce. The NGO workers I observed promoted these animals by emphasizing their commercial value. They offered to link farmers up with commercial vendors servicing provincial markets, and suggested that, if properly raised, the model ducks would be more productive and fetch an equal or higher price than rice-grazing fowl. Such market predictions, however, could not be guaranteed in an economy where the outcome of new livestock varieties and new production regimes remained unknown. As one farm model proponent in Hanoi told me during the planning stages of the intervention, "You know, we should probably check with the guys at the Department of Animal Health to make sure that the models really do increase productivity." Such statements reveal a health programming atmosphere in which the pressure to demonstrate results prompted NGO workers to hurriedly pilot new programs without fully attending to the consequences of their work at intervention sites. In this atmosphere, the success of any one experiment was less important than its ability to generate actionable results.

In fact, productivity and profit did not always surface on model duck farms, because local ecologies and livestock rearing practices pushed against global biosecurity standards. NGO workers found themselves facing frustrated veterinary agents who watched their neighbors lose time, money, and trust in the biosecure system. Hạnh, for instance, did not support the model ducks. She was particularly antagonistic toward Hiển. This stemmed in part from Hiển's overbearing personality but it was also a function of the fact that, in Hạnh's experience, NGO workers like Hiển and Mỹ devised interventions in Ho Chi Minh City and then railroaded them through without regard for local conditions ("what works in An Giang does not necessarily work in Đồng Tháp"). For Hạnh, the NGO representatives were urban interlopers who were more interested in verifying their experiment than promoting farmers' well-being. She told me, "That's how these people work, they go from project to project looking for cash." Hạnh frequently teased the younger Mỹ about her Saigon roots and urban disposition, but left her harsher comments for the elder Hiển. She questioned her knowledge about farming methods and criticized her compassion for farmers. "She doesn't know how to talk to the people. She wants to get all the problems and challenges to report back to [the NGO]. But who's going to sign the biosecurity contract if you are always talking about problems? The farmers are afraid of losses."

Indeed, many farmers had taken a gamble and lost on model varieties. They ended up questioning whether such experimental life forms even belonged in the province. Why did it take so much work for them to survive and grow when free-range ducks got plump simply by picking around in rice paddies? Why don't people want to pay more for infection-free varieties? In this health intervention, the stakes for duck farmers were the same as for any entrepreneur: return on investment. The fact that model ducks could not generate such returns signals a biosecurity apparatus whose outcome is patently *in*-secure.

What distinguishes Naturally Vietnam chickens from model ducks is that they were not expected to outcompete local breeds or commercial varieties, but rather to carve out new markets for traditional yet biosecure life forms. The creation of Naturally Vietnam chickens and the marketing practices surrounding them posited a future of people-poultry exchanges based on biotechnologically enhancing particular designations of "nature" under the auspices of animal health, food safety, and farmer empowerment. The objective of this experiment was twofold. First, it aimed to create value-added chickens that reached biosecurity standards, while simultaneously expressing their primordial, "natural" behaviors. Ideally, these novel life forms would carve out healthy forms of life—nourishing social and ecological relationships with each other, the landscape, and their caretakers. Second, the experiment aimed to increase small farmers' ownership and control over animals from farm to slaughterhouse to market, by creating direct exchange relations between producers and vendors.

When read against model ducks, Naturally Vietnam chickens present a very different kind of entrepreneurial endeavor. The birds were poised to occupy an emerging niche market that catered primarily to expatriate consumers and the small group of elite Vietnamese living among them. It is telling that I met Naturally Vietnam's developer at a high-end restaurant in Hanoi's aptly named "West" Lake district, which is populated by foreign NGOs like CARE International and the World Wildlife Fund, Western restaurant chains like Segafredo Coffee and Al Fresco's, and the opulent houses and apartments of foreign diplomats, NGO workers, financial consultants, and international school teachers. We sampled dishes made from the Naturally Vietnam brand and chatted with the Australian restaurant manager who expressed his commitment to sourcing healthy, low-impact, and sustainable meat for his discerning customers. In addition to this and a few other restaurants, the brand reached consumers at resort hotels in major tourist destinations and at the weekly West Lake open-air market. But achieving such niche market relations was difficult and risky. It required considerable luck and maneuvering. Farmers could only capitalize on the chickens and their elite consumer base if they lived in a province lucky enough to compete for development assistance from the foreign donor, and only if government officials and multinational consultants identified them as appropriate subjects of experimental intervention.

In sum, the life forms and forms of life emerging together in each of these biosecurity experiments were less indicative of clientship than they were of entrepreneurship. Experimental farmers were not clients. They did not come to biosecurity interventions as vulnerable subjects in need of health care. Rather, they were entrepreneurs. Favored by an economization of life in Vietnam that privileges market actors, these entrepreneurs enrolled in experiments as risk-taking businesspersons who demanded returns on their investments. Like the fowl they cultivated, entrepreneurial farmers straddled security and market concerns, and in doing so they engaged in new and uncertain exchange relationships with poultry and other humans.

Conclusion

Whether commercial or traditional, the life forms that surfaced in these experiments belie any proclamation that biosecurity is about preventing flu, *not* promoting economics. On livestock farms, where biological life forms are also commodities, security cannot be divorced from economic considerations. The task of biosecurity interventions has therefore been to generate livestock and production arrangements that can embody these dual considerations. I have shown how experiments to establish flu-free poultry subpopulations also created value-added livestock commodities, which were meant to circulate in distinct ecologies and economies. Such commoditized life forms are still in their trial phases, and their future existence and proliferation depends upon a whole host of factors that start from the level of individual bodies and extend out to global commodity flows.

Yet, their indeterminate status does not mean that these life forms were wholly new, for biosecurity is just one of a long series of on-the-farm biological experiments.[3] Livestock has always been defined by its malleability, and it is no surprise that efforts to securitize these animals are characterized by "indeterminacy and indecision" (Hinchliffe 2001). Farm biosecurity is an emergent, experimental arena that has to weigh what are often conflicting interests against each other, including productivity, security, and health. In Vietnam there are additional interests at play, which include farmer empowerment, the preservation of place and tradition, and the pursuit of poultry happiness. The success of biosecure life forms thus depends upon the extent to which they are able to gain a foothold—compete—in already existing regimes of value.

Model ducks, it turns out, were not very competitive. The biosecurity precepts that limited their mobility had a negative effect on the exchange relations that animated southern delta economies. The enclosures on biosecure farm models restricted poultry movements in order to prevent unsanctioned contact between creatures and ecologies. Such limitations, however, had unintended effects. Duck mobility has traditionally synchronized rice and poultry economies in the south, and ducks and duck farmers have long exhibited an entrepreneurial spirit that brings them into collaboration with different ecological and economic actors. Enclosing ducks in a single space, however, reorganized the kinds and quality of exchange relationships that have long animated the delta region. In promoting biosecure life forms and forms of life, health strategists co-opted the entrepreneurial spirit so characteristic of Mekong Delta residents (Guerrero Blanco 2013) and redirected it into purposefully compartmentalized, commercial transactions. These transactions, however, were not as profitable as promised, and model ducks' failure to compete with local varieties compromised their standing in southern poultry markets. Cultivating this life form hardly seemed worth the risk when at the end of the day farmers' incomes failed to meet, much less surpass, previous levels.

Naturally Vietnam chickens competed within a different regime of value,[4] where the objective was to preserve rather than alter traditional life forms and lifestyles. Everything about these animals was localized. Their branding suggested that they were situated in traditional backyard farms, and their niche marketing limited their circulations to face-to-face, farmer-to-consumer transactions. Naturally Vietnam chickens were less globally ambitious than their model duck counterparts, but in their own way they expanded the purview of global health by appealing not only to disease control but also to matters of tradition and taste. The very name Naturally Vietnam suggests that these life forms were more deeply rooted in notions of place and the values therein, and it is no accident that the chicken developer had lived in Vietnam for many years, spoke the language fluently, and had established a family business in the country. The biosecure form of life he imagined was situated in a sophisticated understanding of and respect for local production practices, chicken sociality, and consumer habits.

But even as it celebrated tradition, the Naturally Vietnam brand occluded a key aspect of "traditional" farming in Vietnam, and that is that backyard chickens are an intentionally low input, low risk, and low investment life form. Even though Naturally Vietnam producers found support from foreign donors, the time, space, and equipment needed to cultivate these disease-free subpopulations required levels of investment and land-use practices that were somewhat at odds with how farmers raise backyard chickens, particularly in the north where space is limited. Also rather untraditional were the types of social relationships and exchanges needed to secure a farmer's place in the very narrow, niche markets in which these animals circulated. These markets were dominated by elite, often foreign urban vendors, whose contact with "traditional" farmers was intermittent at best. Reaching these trading partners required making oneself visible and available to the right people at the right time.

In biosecurity experiments, then, the commoditization of poultry life emerged in conjunction with an economization of life that deemed particular kinds of producers more valuable to the Vietnamese economy. Both of these processes were unsettled. As animals cum commodities cum health therapies, the biosecure life forms described here embodied tensions between the resolutely "public" ethos of global health and the increasingly profit-driven devices of livestock biosecurity. The forms of life required to produce such life forms also embodied these tensions, as model ducks and natural chickens altered multispecies exchange relationships that have long characterized Vietnamese livestock markets. Adopting biosecurity required a risk-taking, entrepreneurial ethos—a willingness to experiment with poultry commodities and people-poultry relationships whose bioeconomic viability and implications remained uncertain.

Hatching

During my time in Placid Pond, I made a habit of accompanying Thủy on her post-siesta walk to her father-in-law's house. She and Trí kept two flocks of hens on Ông Đức's property, and in this daily ritual she collected all their eggs in preparation for Trí's biweekly trip to market. One afternoon, while Thủy was busy in the coops, Ông Đức invited me to have a look at his hatchery. He took me first to the incubation room, which occupied a brick-laid enclosure adjacent to his home. The enclosure was fully one-storey high and about seven feet square, just large enough to fit the hatchery devices and our bodies. It was closed off to the world by a wooden door tied shut with plastic twine, and as soon as we crossed the threshold my senses went to work to adjust to the conditions. It was dark. There were no windows in the enclosure and the lights were turned off, just the sun seeping in from the door we left ajar. It was also warm, even warmer than the late summer tropical temperatures outside. Just to the left of the entrance stood two steel trolleys, about three feet wide, two feet deep and about a foot taller than myself. They faced another pair of trolleys lined up against the opposite wall. Each trolley was lined with open shelves holding trays of eggs. We squeezed into the narrow space between the trolleys. With the heat, the dark, and the stacks and stacks of eggs surrounding us, it was all rather dizzying. Ông Đức focused my attention by removing a tray from its shelf. He explained that the eggs had been incubating for eight days. It would be about ten more before they were ready to hatch.

Ông Đức moved slowly, easing the trays out of metal runners and turning them 180 degrees before sliding them back into place. This rotation process happened once a day, but the trays also needed to be tilted at angles every few hours in order to mimic a hen's brooding process. You could buy shelving units that achieved the tilting automatically, but Ông Đức did this work by hand. Each time he turned the trays, he scanned the eggs with his eyes and nose searching for exploders, a phenomenon in which gas-producing bacteria pops the eggshell and releases a noxious scent and fluid. He selected a few eggs to hold up to the light from the doorway, and showed me how the dim illumination let him assess the embryo's development—her size as well as the position of her head in relation to the shell. I had seen Trí use a stiff rubber tube to inspect an embryo before, placing it against the eggshell and peering through to achieve the same effect. Ông Đức handed me an egg and asked if I could feel the thickness of the shell. Besides its warmth, it didn't feel much different than the unfertilized eggs I picked up at the market, or the ones that Thủy collected from her hens, but Ông Đức explained that the shells were getting thinner and softer, closer to being penetrable by the chick's nascent beak.

There was a thermometer hanging from one of the trolleys but I didn't see Ông Đức consult it. He told me that the temperature should be just about 40 degrees Celsius, like the warmest days of summer. If it got too warm, he opened the door for a time; too cold, and he raised the temperature on the space heater. It should also be humid, but not so humid that it could stunt the embryo's growth—an outcome that Ông Đức said he could feel by the weight of the egg. He added that the embryos are much more sensitive to temperature and humidity in the early days, but as they develop they release their own heat, which must be again accommodated by adjusting the conditions in the incubation room.

When the eggs were ready to hatch, Ông Đức and his wife, Bà An, worked together to transfer them to large, freestanding woven baskets in another brick enclosure. Like incubating, hatching is an exacting process. There must be more ventilation than in the incubator, and the hatching room had small openings in the bricks near the ceiling. There were fans in this room, which kept air flowing and the humidity down, since chicks are in greatest danger of dehydration right before they are about to come into the world. Above each basket hung a heat-emitting light bulb to entice further growth and shell penetration. Inside, unshucked rice grains reached two-thirds of the way to the brim. Here, on the grains, the couple gently placed egg after egg. This required a light touch; pushing the eggs down into the grain would only crack the shell or effect an uneven distribution of temperature. The rice grains provided enough weight and stability to keep the eggs from rolling into one another, but had enough give for minute movements.

The couple left the eggs alone in the baskets; by this time the chicks were ready to do what they needed to on their own. Within a day or two, little chicks would poke their beaks through the top of their eggs, shake off their shells, and stand somewhat dazed under the warmth of the lamp (perhaps looking for their absent mother). This is when Bà An took a more prominent role in the process, looking in on the chicks periodically to make sure they were drinking their nutritive fluid and checking for illness or malformations. A day or two after hatching, Ông Đức's clients would come by the house to buy some chicks to start their own production cycles. Many of his buyers had been transacting with him for decades, while others had just started farming operations with savings from work abroad. Bà An would bring any remaining chicks to one of three neighborhood markets, walking them over in rice baskets suspended from her shoulder pole.

Earlier, I noted that Ông Đức built his chicken hatchery in response to restrictive agricultural governance policies begun at end of the Second Indochina War, and that it has served as a key source of his family's income and social status ever since. Here I have dwelt on the mundane, exacting work of actually bringing chicks out of their shell and into the world, because I want to point to the fact that Ông Đức's hatchery is much more than a maneuver to make do. In the daily work of hatching, Ông Đức attuned his body and his senses to the developing bodies of chicks, caring for them in ways that cannot be captured in strictly economic or political terms.

Care has become an important concept for scholarship that resists viewing animals instrumentally, in terms of the purpose they serve for humans. Early studies of human-animal relations in anthropology took such an instrumental view, and were keen to show that seemingly curious cosmological beliefs and ritual behaviors surrounding animals actually served important ecological and political-economic functions—whether in the economically adaptive Hindu prohibition against consuming cows in India (Harris 1974), the ecosystemic equilibrium achieved by ritual pig slaughter in New Guinea (Rappaport 1967), or the "mutually parasitic" systems in which Nuer people raise cattle who in turn provide alimentary resources, insurance against hazards, and exchange goods for creating sociopolitical bonds among people and the divine (Evans-Pritchard 1940, 36). More recently, anthropologists have elaborated on these approaches by replacing questions about what animals do for humans with questions about how animals relate to humans in patterned and meaningful social arrangements—forms of life (Baynes-Rock 2015; Kirksey 2014; Nading 2014a; Ogden 2011; Parrenas 2012; Tsing 2015). To do so, they often focus on bodies—life forms—and explore the sites and moments in which human and nonhuman animals corporeally perceive, respond to, and affect one another. Such bodily exchanges are more than instrumental; they create affinities, connections, and shared understandings across species (Despret 2004; Haraway 2007).

These bodily exchanges also have health consequences. Medical anthropologists have long argued that health and well-being are a social pheno-
mena that rests on the cultivation of mutually affective and responsive bodily
interactions (Csordas 2011; Farquhar and Lock 2007; Gammeltoft 2008;
Scheper-Hughes and Lock 1987). This is true for human as well as multispecies communities (Blanchette 2018; Gruen 2014; Porter 2018; Weaver
2013). Vinciane Despret has shown that the most successful human-animal
pairings are those in which participants allow themselves to be shaped by
others, bodily and otherwise (Despret 2004, 115). Despret calls these relationships of care. Care is an ethical obligation and a practical process that requires
getting concretely involved in looking after another (Bellacasa 2012, 197). It
involves immersing yourself in the multitude of problems presented by another, and allowing them to express things that might not meet your expectations (Despret 2004, 128). Care is a process of coming to agreement, whereby
different beings negotiate and tinker with their unique ways of perceiving
and experiencing the world (Mol 2008). The form that care takes is therefore open-ended, and it's not always clear who is in control. In multispecies
relationships, care is also risky; it means becoming vulnerable and realizing
that vulnerability is unequally distributed across different life forms (Parrenas 2012, 682).

Ông Đức's hatching practices reflected these concepts of care. He exposed
himself to the embryos' environment and calibrated his body to share in and
enrich their world. Making his senses available to the embryos allowed him
to make concrete adjustments, to tinker, in ways that aided in their development. Both Ông Đức and the chicks were affected by this process. Hatching
followed particular, human-directed patterns and principles, but it required
maintenance, in which different the life forms read and responded to one another with their bodies. Embryonic chicks' physiological experiences and expressions shaped Ông Đức's own experiences and expressions, and vice versa.
Put simply, care was not a unidirectional human intervention into poultry
bodies. Instead, it was a kind of partnership in which person and poultry
became immersed in one another.

While Ông Đức's hatching practices appeared coordinated and harmoni-
ous, other embryo exchanges display care's contingency and violence. Thủy
was pregnant with her second child when I lived with her family in Placid
Pond. Early on in the pregnancy, we were eating soup when Trí pointed to a
duck embryo in the broth and announced that we must save it for Thủy. Thủy
said that the duck embryo floating in the soup was like the human embryo
gestating in her womb, and just as the amniotic fluids in the egg provide
nutrients to growing duck, so they would for her growing baby. This identity

between human and avian life forms meant that eating the duck embryo would transfer its vitality and fertility to Thủy's embryo at a particularly vulnerable stage in her pregnancy.[1] In addition to illustrating fluid boundaries between bodies, Thủy's consumption practices offer a salient example of the ways that care distributes risk and vulnerability unequally. Though mundane, this act reminds us that killing and care are braided together in everyday exchanges between species (Doreen 2014; Bellacasa 2012). Difference and inequality continue to matter in relationships of care, and in communities where people and poultry live together, human health and well-being often rule the day.

Taken together, these forms of care reveal how bodily exchanges provide diverse opportunities for mutual discovery and transformation. But they also raise questions about how we comport our own bodies in the presence of other species, and about how we should intervene in the bodies of others (Chiew 2014; Gruen 2014; Greenhough and Roe 2011; Rock and Degeling 2015). I want to keep these questions in mind as I turn my attention back to bird flu experiments. As I work through these experiments, I ask, which exchanges encourage us to live well with others in a pandemic age? And, is it possible to do better?

Enumerating Immunity

Bring pandemics up in any conversation and you will almost certainly hit on the topic of vaccination, one of the most common, and controversial, methods for addressing infectious diseases. Common because vaccination offers a quick, technical fix that can impart immunity at the individual and population levels. Controversial because limited supplies make it difficult to ethically distribute vaccines to ensure equal access, especially in cases where pathogens transcend national borders and socioeconomic divisions. In 2014, health officials ran into problems when they tried to run on-the-ground tests of experimental Ebola vaccines, as questions about who should be immunized in the midst of outbreaks loomed large. The same questions appeared again during the spread of Zika virus the following year. Vaccine controversies only heighten when the prospect of profit is thrown into the mix. The development of both H5N1 and H1N1 influenza vaccines sparked accusations that commercial pharmaceutical interests were dictating where and when vaccines would appear—and, for whom.

While these controversies have largely centered on human inoculations, in the case of infections that cross species it is also important to pay attention to animal vaccines. One Health programs for zoonoses and vector-borne diseases are increasingly experimenting with ways to neutralize the pathogenic potential of *animal* hosts and vectors as a means to protect humans from exposure (Biesel and Boete 2013; Fearnley 2018; Kelly and Lezaun 2013 Nading 2014a, 2014b). This is certainly true for Vietnam and other bird flu-affected countries, where HPAI vaccines target poultry rather than people. Problems of equitable access and distribution take new form in these settings, as public health agendas to protect human lives rub up against commercial agendas to protect poultry commodities. With livestock as the subject of bodily intervention, new questions arise, not only about who gets vaccines, but also about who gets to administer them, thereby bringing new actors and interests into the realm of global health governance.

I now turn to mass poultry vaccination, an unverified, experimental bird flu strategy that seeks to mitigate the risk of human infection by reducing the viruses circulating in poultry. Though vaccination targets poultry biology, its effects span far beyond the organic realm to impact social and economic arrangements in farming communities. I want to know how these prophylactic interventions into poultry bodies end up changing the actors and practices involved in livestock care more broadly, and I want to know how these changes affect communities where humans live most closely with animals. To answer these questions, I trace how poultry vaccines circulate on the ground, in everyday exchanges between state veterinarians, farmers, and fowl. I begin by describing the inoculation activities of state veterinarians. Following veterinarians' daily routines shows that in a national context of scarce resources and the privatization of health services, state veterinarians distribute vaccine supplies in uneven ways. In turn, such spotty distribution prompts farmers to protect their flocks by other means, and in accordance with their own assessments of bird flu risks in relation to other threats, biological and otherwise. I then go on to describe farmers' vaccination strategies. I argue that programs meant to protect humans through the immunization of birds find little purchase in settings where HPAI inordinately affects poultry, and where policy makers, veterinarians, and farmers have different priorities surrounding the protection and valuation of different lives and livelihoods. Taken together, the stories I share here reveal that when pandemic vaccines target animals, questions about access are as much about rights to commodities as they are about rights to health; and questions about distribution are as much about expertise (in other words, who is equipped to inoculate animals) and risk (i.e., which diseases people and poultry are most vulnerable to) as they are about equity.

By the time poultry vaccination measures were implemented in 2005, "Vietnam faced a public health crisis" (Sims and Do 2009). The country sat near the top of the worldwide list of reported human and poultry cases, with numbers continuing to rise. Traditional zoonoses control measures such as culling, disinfection, and movement control were failing to prevent outbreaks among animals and humans.[1] With fears of a pandemic rising, health strategists turned to less conventional, and more experimental, methods to address HPAI. The NSCAI's first Integrated National Plan for Avian Influenza Control and Human Pandemic Preparedness and Response (2006–8), known popularly as "The Red Book," explains the rationale behind mass poultry vaccination. It highlights the uncertainty against which vaccination emerges:

> The world is concerned about the possible emergence of a strain of influenza capable of transmitting directly from human to human. The risk of this occurring increases with the number of human exposures. NSCAI considered it extremely important to reduce the amount of circulating virus and therefore the likelihood of exposure of people to these viruses . . . the use of vaccination was seen as a valuable tool for reducing human (and poultry) exposure (National Steering Committee on Human and Avian Influenza 2006b, 16).

This statement highlights a few key aspects of poultry vaccination as an experiment in One Health governance. First, vaccination focuses in on the H5N1 virus itself as the problem that needs to be addressed — more specifically, the particular strain of H5N1 virus circulating in Vietnamese poultry. Under the right (unknown) conditions, this strain could jump species to infect humans, and even mutate to achieve human-to-human transmission. Poultry vaccination, though untested, is seen as a way to stave off such impending mutations. Second, vaccination conceives of poultry as a viral reservoir. Here, the avian body becomes available for prophylactic intervention primarily *as a means to protect humans*. Poultry health is quite literally a parenthetical consideration in this strategy. Third, vaccination offers a targeted, biological approach that bypasses the ecological, social, and economic conditions of virus emergence and spread. It effectively decontextualizes the virus from its social relations with hosts and habitats. Put another way, vaccination separates life forms from forms of life, altering one experimental variable while attempting to hold the other in place.

Early on, policy makers recognized the limits of such a targeted, technical approach to disease control. From the very beginning, national leaders proposed vaccination as a short-term measure to introduce alongside long-term structural and ecological transformations to livestock economies. The NSCAI's second Integrated National Plan for Avian Influenza Control and Human Pandemic Preparedness and Response (2006–10), known popularly as "The Green Book," states:

> The current vaccination program is seen as the first phase in a long-term program to control and eventually eliminate H5N1 HPAI from Viet Nam. Vaccination is being used at present to dampen down the levels of infection, providing an opportunity to implement some of the structural changes needed to assist in control. . . . Vaccination will be required for some years to come as an aid in controlling avian influenza in Viet Nam, but the intensive blanket program, as currently practiced, cannot be sustained for very long (National Steering Committee on Human and Avian Influenza 2006c, 19).

Here, the NSCAI further elaborates the experimental, future-oriented ethos of poultry vaccination. This statement weaves vaccination into a patchwork of strategies for pandemic planning and establishes linear, temporal continuity between the technical fix and farther-reaching transformations in Vietnam's livestock sector. Delineating vaccination as a "first phase" step to "dampen down levels of infection" permits policy makers to limit their response to the virus itself, while still acknowledging the broader aims and timelines of HPAI governance.

Yet, in spite of rhetoric about its inbuilt impermanence, over ten years on vaccination remains a primary avian flu control strategy in Vietnam (and some other affected countries), in part because virtually no avian or human HPAI outbreaks have been traced back to vaccinated flocks.[2] The country's continued reliance on what was meant to be a short-term measure has aggravated some health workers on the ground. A senior transnational epidemiologist in Hanoi explained it this way:

> A strategy against the virus is not enough; you've also got to consider the environment, people, animals, genetics, and immunology. Vaccination of humans is the best option. An animal vaccine is different; it's not complete and not sustainable. We don't know which virus will cause a pandemic. . . . People implement a policy that's not agreed upon, or they see that a policy isn't working but don't say anything. It's driven by a need to maintain control, to not let the population panic.

This is a strong statement against Vietnam's first-line defense against HPAI, one that reveals the contingency of such a flu control program. Frankly, I was surprised to hear it coming from a long-time global health worker and Hanoi resident. Of course, a few other experts had also critiqued poultry vaccination. But their criticisms were more in line with NSCAI statements that recognized its positive impact on outbreaks while expressing concern about long-term costs to the nation. This epidemiologist, however, went so far as to say that vaccination wasn't working. What did he mean by this? If there were quantifiable outbreak reductions, how was the vaccination intervention failing? I decided to find out by looking at vaccination in practice.

Inoculation, In Situ

Highly pathogenic avian influenza vaccines surfaced within a Vietnamese animal health system that had raised concerns about whether local veterinarians could adequately respond to the virus. "Strengthening national veterinary services" and "building national veterinary capacity" were oft-repeated phrases in both official and unofficial rhetoric at the time of my research. As part of efforts to bolster animal health, the NSCAI elected to implement poultry vaccinations through the arm of state veterinarians, including (1) *cán bộ thú y* (veterinary cadres, or state-employed provincial, district, and commune-level vets); and (2) *thú y viên* (paraveterinary workers, or semi-professional animal health workers trained and employed by the state to assist in disease-control measures). In practice, this has meant that state-employed veterinarians have shouldered the responsibility of seasonally vaccinating Vietnam's entire poultry population for over a decade. This is a monumental task, and something I observed firsthand during research with district-level veterinarians in Đồng Tháp province.

One day of vaccination sticks out as particularly memorable. It was late summer, the rainy season, and the first day of the workweek. At around 7:00 in the morning I parked my motorbike at the threshold of a storefront featuring an array of livestock medications, feed, and equipment. The store belonged to Mai, a district veterinarian, shop owner, and pig farmer. After selling a kilogram of chicken feed and a few packages of antibiotic to a young woman, Mai sat down next to me, ordered two iced coffees from the vendor next door, and picked up the phone. In quick succession she called four duck farmers and her two apprentices Toàn and Hưng. "9:30. Green Leaf Village. Five hundred ducks," she said, announcing our first appointment.

The late-morning appointment gave Mai enough time to stop by her hog farm and clean out the sties. She threw a twenty-five-kilo sack of feed over her five-foot frame and picked up her sunglasses. "You drive," she told me, and as we mounted the motorbike she positioned the bag between our bodies. The added, unresponsive weight on bike took some getting used to, but Mai helped me navigate the bumpiest bits, moving the sack along with her body to correspond with the bike's own momentum. When we arrived at the farm we woke up Mai's father-in-law, whose job it was to sleep at the farm in order to guard the animals. Mai led me to the concrete sties out back. There were four in total and they housed the largest hogs I have ever seen. No Vietnamese pot-bellied pigs or beatific Babes here. As we passed each enclosure, Mai told me about her recent investment in the farm, the costs of putting up the sties and paying for the industrial feed, and the price she hoped to get for the hogs once they went to market.

Although the pigs promised added income, Mai complained that they took time away from her storefront business as well as her veterinary work. "You see how I had to close down the shop to do this, and in the morning when people are doing all their shopping!" I sympathized, even more so when I came to see how unpleasant pig farming is. Mai handed me a hose about five inches in diameter, which propelled me forward when she turned it on. My body was taxed under the volume of the water, and I was frankly terrified of the animals. Over three times my weight, the hogs glared and snarled as I pointed the hose their way, and they feigned (?) attack when I got too close. The water released a noxious stench as it washed away the urine and feces, which, when added to the heat and glare of the morning sun, made my head spin. I felt relieved, and a bit guilty, when the time came to meet Toàn and Hưng for the poultry vaccination.

Getting to the first duck farm required taking a ferry across a river, parking our motorbikes at a café (several plastic chairs arranged under a tarpaulin canopy), and walking half a mile over rice paddies muddied by the seasonal rains. My footing had improved over the last few weeks but I still managed to slip and catch a toenail on a rock. Toàn, ever vigilant, prevented my fall. Sandals were more treacherous than bare feet on this terrain. When we reached the farm gate, we were told that Ông Chính forgot we were coming and already took his ducks out to feed. We would have to come back at 4:00. Backtracking, Mai called out to the neighboring farmer, asking if he'd vaccinated his flocks yet. No, he explained. He did last year but they didn't need it because there weren't any outbreaks.

"You should!" she prodded.

"*Mai sau,* later on."

Mai sighed. It was not compulsory for farmers to vaccinate at the time I was in Đồng Tháp (because there were no active outbreaks in the country) but it was in Mai's interest to document as many vaccinations as possible for the District Zoonoses Committee. After all, according to provincial policy she would be fined if an outbreak occurred in an unvaccinated flock. Though she was frustrated, Mai understood the farmer's position. As we walked back to the motorbikes she explained that many farmers, particularly those with small flocks, were wary of vaccines. Some animals became lethargic, ill, or even died after being vaccinated, and of course it was difficult not to draw a connection between inoculation and illness.

We had better luck with the farmer down the way who said we could vaccinate his chickens, a rarity in this duck-driven economy. Donning their pristine white lab coats, latex gloves, and face masks, Toàn and Hưng removed the vaccine bottles from their handheld cooler, attached gun-shaped steel syringes to the tops, and placed the bottles in their pockets. With these accoutrements the assistants appeared to stand more erect and to move with more precision. I had begun to think of these materials and devices as more than tools of the trade; they seemed to discipline the veterinarians' bodies and mark their medical authority. I guessed that this was why I was given a lab coat when I began working with the team, and why I was instructed to spend my evenings washing it by hand.

There were fewer than fifty chickens on this farm, so Mai didn't offer to help. Instead she answered a call requesting her to vaccinate a litter of piglets in her commune. She promised to stop by at 3:00. Twenty minutes later the apprentices had finished the task and we began making our way to the next farm. But after just a few kilometers of slow driving, Hưng's bike got stuck in the mud and it took three of us to push it out. At any rate we couldn't use the bikes for long. Getting to the next farm required navigating a wooden skiff through several small canals. Mai rowed while Toàn jumped in and out of the vessel to remove debris and foliage blocking our path.

By the time we arrived at the farm the sun was high in the sky and sweat was collecting on our foreheads. The farm owner, Ông Cương, had fourteen hundred ducks and it was their first round of vaccine. The job would require all of our hands as well as the assistance of Ông Cương and his seasonal employees. Ông Cương was intrigued my participation and lobbed lewd comments my way: "Be gentle with that probe, it's his first time." Despite the joke, I noticed that he noticed how I was holding the birds. Every few minutes, and with a cautionary glance, he would reposition a duck in my hands to avoid bruising their neck. His neighbor stopped by to join the activity and to chide Mai about his flock. "I called you last week to vaccinate but you weren't around." Mai explained that she was attending a meeting in the provincial capital (a meeting on how to share HPAI reports between communes). "What a pain," he said, "And now my ducks are out grazing."

A few minutes into the job the afternoon rains began, making it difficult for me to see if the needle was driving into the right spot. Hưng explained that it wasn't so much a matter of seeing than feeling the needle punch through the skin of the forehead. But I was having trouble paying attention. I was troubled by the fact that the birds' thrashing had already shredded my "protective" latex gloves, and I wondered what infections I could pick up if they broke through my skin. Animal agency indeed. Ông Cương picked up a bird and guided my hands to the chest. "Here's where you want it, feel the meaty part here. It'd be just my luck to have a flu outbreak because the American 'expert' messed up!" One of the hired farmhands who had been observing carefully asked for my syringe and started injecting the ducks himself. Mai didn't seem to mind and I was frankly glad to just catch and hand over the birds rather than try to maneuver a needle while they squirmed, kicked, and bashed me with their wings. It seemed that anybody could administer vaccine; no technical experience or training required.

After we had injected every bird, Mai bent over the mini cooler filled with

serum in order to fill out the immunization certificate, which by then had
been thoroughly soiled by rain, blood, and vaccine. The rest of us washed our
hands in the river where we had just released the ducks. Soap, another first
defense against the virus, eluded us. It was now 3:30 and I for one was starv-
ing. But there was no time to eat. Toàn, Hưng, and I had to go back to Ông
Chính's farm, and Mai had to immunize those piglets. "Get more vaccine,
we're running out," Mai yelled to her apprentices. Another few canal rides
and two hundred ducks later, we arrived back to the store just as the sun was
setting. Bruised, bloodied, wet, and exhausted, all I wanted was dinner and a
bath. But the team had other plans. Hưng took off to the veterinary office to
refrigerate what was left of the vaccine. Toàn ran the storefront so that Mai
could submit the immunization records to the People's Committee. I helped
Mai's daughter with her math homework.

Though I was exhausted, I was also invigorated by all the activity. When
she returned, I asked Mai whether I should come by the next morning.

"No, there's not enough vaccine," she said. "The next batch comes next
week."

In recounting this day, I am reminded of the incredible stamina that it
takes for veterinarians to inoculate in their jurisdictions. Vietnam is a hot

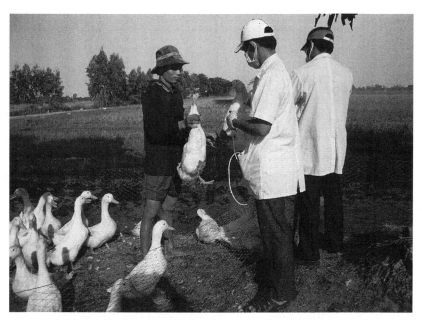

FIG. 3. H5N1 vaccination on a semi-commercial duck farm in Đồng Tháp province. District veterinarians, Hưng and Toàn, inject the birds while a farmhand gathers and presents them for inoculation. Photo
by author.

and wet place; the sun saps your energy, and the rain compromises your senses. The terrain in the southern delta region is unpredictable; a road one day could be a flooded bog the next. And the animals are unruly. Like their owners, they do not appreciate the advances of veterinarians into their space, and my bruised and bloodied arms revealed that they are even less receptive to preventative probes. The work of poultry vaccination also reveals the chancy, often violent bodily encounters involved in animal care (Haraway 2007; Giraud and Hollin 2016). In her study of orangutan conservation in Malaysia, Juno Parrenas describes how caring for animals is a laborious process that brings bodies into close, intimate contact with one another. This labor is risky, but Parrenas shows that the risks are always unequally distributed between the different species involved (2012, 674). Like conservation, vaccination is a form of labor that brings species together into intimate, risky bodily exchanges. And, like conservation, these risks are also unequally distributed across different bodies. In the work of immunizing, Mai, Toàn, Hưng were protected from the causes and consequences of virus emergence in ways that farmers were not. Their bodily encounters with ducks were structured by layers of protection—lab coats, face masks, gloves—devices and safeguards that were unavailable to the farmers who were also engaged in the work of inoculation. Besides these biological invulnerabilities, vets also enjoyed a layer of economic protection. Although Mai was fined if an outbreak of HPAI occurred in an unvaccinated flock in her jurisdiction, that financial loss paled in comparison to the losses farmers suffered as a result of poultry infection and the mandatory culling measures that followed. Ông Cường recognized these inequities and chose to insert himself into the inoculation process, watching our movements carefully and sharing his expertise. The ducks, of course, were the most vulnerable; their necks were grasped, their bodies jerked upward, and their throats were squeezed tightly. All of this only to be stuck with an injection meant to protect, but also known to stun, weaken, and sometimes even kill them.

Yet still, veterinarians were not entirely immune to risks. In recounting this day, I am also reminded of some of the structural forces that make vets vulnerable in the work of vaccination. Shortages of state-supplied serum and the requirements of auxiliary work commitments made it difficult for veterinarians to keep appointments to inoculate flocks, and as such deterred farmers from relying on them to allocate or administer vaccines. In fact, many farmers I spoke to told me that they avoided vaccination since they were never sure if state vets actually had the vaccine; and even if they did, the vaccine might be expired or defective. State veterinarians like Mai complained that they were in competition with other provinces for vaccines, and that they

often had to wait several months for delivery. In addition to vaccine shortages, Mai and her colleagues were also embedded in a livestock economy in
which a variety of other animals competed with poultry for veterinary attention. Mai literally ran from farm to farm, splitting her time among pigs,
poultry, fish, and the occasional cow or water buffalo. When coupled with
the scarcity of vaccines, veterinarians' responsibilities to these other livestock
(including those they owned themselves) compromised their ability to carry
out their jobs, eroded what standing they had in their communities, and put
them at risk for public scorn and financial penalty.

Privatizing Probes

The difficulties that state veterinarians like Mai faced when trying to vaccinate poultry in her jurisdiction were not simply an issue of difficult terrain,
recalcitrant bodies, or limited resources. They also had to do with ambigui-
ties about whether state agents were in the best position to care for livestock,
particularly in a veterinary sector where animal care is carried out by a variety of actors with varied experience. In Vietnam, HPAI vaccines circulate
in an animal health system in which unregulated private practitioners and
veterinary pharmaceutical retailers have become ubiquitous. These providers
cater especially to rural dwellers who not only lack the funds for increasingly
for-fee public services, but also lack the means to travel to public providers
and certified drug retailers (Nguyen et al. 2008; Chaudhuri and Roy 2008). A
comprehensive report on Vietnam's veterinary sector compiled by the World
Organization for Animal Health (OIE) concluded that public veterinarians
work alongside private veterinarians, paravets, and drug shop retailers. "All
of them seem to be allowed to undertake any type of activity," and the lack of
coordination among these actors has hampered efforts to launch a sustainable vaccination program (Fermet-Quinet, Jane, and Forman 2007, 83).

Farmers' lack of enthusiasm for state-administered vaccination can be at-
tributed in part to the lack of clarity surrounding veterinary authority, but a
bigger deterrent is the fact that farmers themselves have historically carried
out this work. Given its long history and geographic pervasiveness in Vietnam, farmers usually talked about poultry keeping as a matter of common
sense, not professional expertise. One of the phrases I heard most often when
asking farmers about their poultry keeping activities was, "I just do what's
normal (*bình thường*)," a statement that highlights the ordinary, unexceptional nature of poultry care. When farmers did turn to vets, it was largely
in their capacity as private drug retailers, rather than state-employed animal health professionals. Mai conducted a swift private drug trade from her

storefront, and most of the time her customers not only knew what medications they wanted, but they also administered them themselves. Put another way, poultry have long enjoyed a level of immunity from state intervention.

Multinational strategists have responded to hiccups in the state provision of vaccines by suggesting measures to privatize HPAI inoculations. Privatization, they argue, would be more natural in a context where farmers largely avoid state veterinary services anyway. In 2008, Andrew Speedy of the FAO in Vietnam made a speech in a "Meeting to Review the Strategy for Control and Prevention of Highly Pathogenic Avian Influenza in the Agriculture Sector." He stated:

> Public-private cost sharing will not only enable the governments at the central, provincial and district levels to have some budgetary reserves for supporting other key disease prevention and control interventions, but is also likely to bring about a sense of ownership and therefore stronger participation in the vaccination policy by all those involved in the poultry business (Speedy 2008, "Speech").

This excerpt was included in a joint WHO, FAO, and OIE report entitled, "Vietnam's New AI Strategy." Deploying concepts of "ownership" and "participation," the report justified reductions in government spending through a discourse that brought public health under the remit of private, commercial activity. But reductions in government spending are still reductions in government spending, and medical anthropologist João Biehl has observed that rhetoric about public-private mixtures adds a moral spin on what is essentially a tenet of neoclassical economics: a self-regulating market (2006, 208).

Public-private cost sharing ultimately means transferring responsibilities for health care from states to citizens and for-profit actors. In Vietnam, this transfer of responsibilities is made possible by the fact that bird flu surfaces in livestock economies. By casting public-private cost sharing as a matter of "poultry business," *not* public health, multinational strategists effectively shift the objective of vaccine interventions from safeguarding human life to protecting commodity investments. Inasmuch as poultry are by definition livestock, it seems reasonable to claim that responsibility for their life and health falls to private citizens rather than public health workers. And so by positing an approach to epidemics that is *poultry-*, not people-, centered, "Vietnam's new AI strategy" removes the state (and its multinational supporters) from the rubric of health provision. And so even though mass poultry vaccination was introduced as a means to stave off human infection, as the experiment proceeded, the targets and beneficiaries of inoculation shifted.

What I want to highlight here is that when the target of flu control shifts to livestock, and responsibility from states to citizens, a whole host of added interests and vulnerabilities are brought into play in bird flu governance. The fact that Mai divided her workday among poultry, pigs, and other livestock shows that bird flu vaccines circulate in a bioeconomy of agricultural production in which H5N1 is only one of a range of pathogens, and poultry is only one of a range of differently valued livestock commodities. In spite of all the international attention, avian flu is a low priority for farmers and veterinarians alike, and it is telling that Mai chose to invest in a hog farm to supplement her income, and that she left the work of poultry vaccination to her apprentices while she set off to inoculate piglets.

The time I spent with Hương, a district veterinarian in Bắc Giang, further illustrated how different species are valued in the everyday provision of animal health. Though I had hoped to observe her inoculating chickens, I found myself at countless pig farms, vaccinating, castrating, and cutting the fangs off of tiny piglets. Hương explained that she vaccinated pigs far more frequently than poultry because the loss of time and income from the death of a pig outweighs that of a chicken or duck many times over. In light of such risks, farmers were not only more concerned with vaccinating large animals; they were also willing to pay Hương for the service. Like Mai down south, Hương spent her time keeping abreast of the latest pharmaceutical developments and health issues related to large livestock so that she could effectively treat these animals, for a fee.

But in concentrating on the health of large livestock, state veterinarians compromised their standing among poultry farmers, who often underlined their ignorance with regard to poultry. Inasmuch as district and commune level veterinarians undergo one year or less of formal training (with paravets and apprentices receiving even less), most farmers considered their intelligence and education level to be sub-par. Compounding this educational dearth, veterinarians' decision to focus their attention on large livestock meant that farmers often exercised vigilance with state administered poultry inoculation, or else sought vaccination services elsewhere. Working alongside Mai revealed that many farmers scrutinized how vets interacted with poultry, and made suggestions about how to handle, position, and probe their birds. Some particularly scrupulous farmers went so far as to describe the proclivities and habits of their specific birds to vets, and asked them to vaccinate in a particular place on poultry bodies to avoid ill effects. Still other farmers refused vaccination altogether.

A vocal minority of global health workers tried to give voice to tensions about which life forms deserve consideration in Vietnamese livestock economies. These individuals recognized that H5N1 viruses exist alongside a range of other biological threats in Vietnam, only some of which infect humans, but all of which impact the health, productivity, and marketability of animal commodities. One notable agitator was Kim, an Australian veterinarian employed by the WHO. Kim's placement in the WHO was part of a multinational strategy to address zoonoses by inserting veterinary expertise into global health programming. In our first meeting, however, Kim complained that global health and development workers were paying too much attention to bird flu. Even though her position was established as a result of HPAI funding, she had decided to focus her work on "neglected zoonoses." When I asked why, she said:

> They're all working on AI [avian influenza]. . . . I don't like the hype around these diseases. In fact, there are many other diseases that impact people. For example, Newcastle disease here, which shares many of the same symptoms with AI. There's an effective vaccine for this disease, which has a significant impact on poultry. But Newcastle is here; it doesn't affect the whole world.

Kim's frustration with bird flu signals a broader trend in global health governance, in which multinational donors and agencies prioritize "global" risks over more pressing domestic ones (Janes and Corbett 2009; Pfeiffer and Nichter 2008). But by locating bird flu viruses in a local ecology in which they circulate alongside a number of other pathogens, Kim brought different interests into the fold of One Health programming. Her specific example of Newcastle disease is important here. Newcastle infection spreads quickly and easily among poultry flocks and results in significant poultry deaths and financial losses for farmers. Quantitative studies and my own observations suggest that poultry producers are more concerned with preventing Newcastle disease than H5N1 (CARE International Vietnam 2006; Otte 2007), and many farmers who chose not to vaccinate their flocks for avian flu willingly paid out of pocket for the Newcastle vaccine. As one farmer related to me, "We've never seen bird flu here, but Newcastle is all over the place. The chickens become sick and die very quickly." But even though Newcastle devastates farmers' source of income and protein, outside of the rare case of mild flu it does not compromise their immune systems. The virus's effects on humans are more socioeconomic than biological, more local than global.

Put simply, H5N1 viruses circulate in economies where they compete with other livestock pathogens. And so when HPAI vaccines began circulating in these same economies, they generated conflicts among people who expressed different ways of assessing viruses, and different ways of caring for livestock. In what follows, I consider these conflicts from the vantage point of poultry farmers.

Kinship, Control, and Care

Recall that the rationale behind poultry vaccination is that immunizing poultry will protect against the emergence of a human pandemic virus. But in fact many farmers suggested that the frequency and proximity with which they interfaced with poultry actually already prevented human infection, and they themselves were not worried about contracting bird flu. These farmers were nevertheless eager to vaccinate against bird flu; they just did so in order to protect poultry health (Tran et al. 2006). Trí explained to me that "all of the diseases, Gumboro, Marek, Newcastle, bird flu, are really important so we have to vaccinate for all of them. We mostly do them our selves, you know. The veterinarians don't help the people. If we don't, the chickens will die early on." When I asked about human infection, he responded, "People dying? People can't get sick from chickens. . . . We can't catch bird flu."

Corporeal contact is not only a source of human immunity to bird flu. It also forms the foundation of poultry care. Donna Haraway (2007) suggests that it is through the act of touch that multispecies actors learn to care for and become response-able to one another. Through touch, different life forms recognize each other and their mutual dependencies. For Trí and his neighbors, the reoccurring and mundane patterns of contact between people and poultry conferred a responsibility to guard against a *range* of infections in order to protect their poultry and their livelihoods. In contrast to official rhetoric, then, poultry health was not a parenthetical concern for farmers like Trí, but rather the main priority and objective of vaccination strategies. Seen from this vantage point, the work of caring for poultry fell to farmers, those who had more skin in the game (literally and figuratively).

Early on in my fieldwork in Placid Pond I observed Thủy and Trí carry out a Newcastle vaccination. It was obvious from the beginning that job was a family affair. After a quick dinner, I accompanied Trí, Thủy, and their daughter, Qui, to Ông Đức's house. I sat down with the kids in the courtyard, eating green mangoes and chatting with Ông Đức as he smoked from a water pipe. We watched as Trí retrieved the vaccine from his father's refrigerator and brought it over to one of the coops where Thủy was cordoning off about two hundred birds with a blue tarpaulin. After the sun had fully set, Trí's teenage neighbor arrived, followed soon after by Trí's bellowing cousin Mịnh, who immediately set upon teasing the women present.

Following a smoke and some greetings, everyone got to work. We entered the coop where the birds stood behind the tarp, quiet because of the dark and their confinement. After shaking the vaccine and pouring it into a rice bowl, Trí set up a plastic chair on which he placed the solution and two syringes. He told Qui and their neighbor to squat next to the chair and showed them how to measure the solution to the spot he had marked on the syringe. This was serious business. Trí was visibly tense and the young girls worked with exacting care. Trí then joined Mịnh in a squatting position opposite Ông Đức, ready to grasp the birds that Thủy and Trí's mother would hand over to them. The women were stationed behind the tarp where they sidled up next to the birds, stooped down, grabbed their legs, and flipped them upside down. After collecting three birds, they hung each batch over the tarp and waited for Trí and Mịnh to grab them. In a fluid collection of movements, Trí received the birds with his left hand, steadied them with his right, and placed them down in front of his father who plunged the syringe into their breasts. Trí then swept the inoculated fowl to the side and lifted his arms toward Thủy, who handed him another set of feet. He never looked up; he just felt for the birds. Meanwhile, Mịnh placed another batch of birds in front of Ông Đức. Every twenty or so rounds of inoculation, Ông Đức requested more vaccine from the girls.

The process lasted about forty minutes and by the end everyone was stiff and sweaty. The immunization went off without a hitch, though. It was a

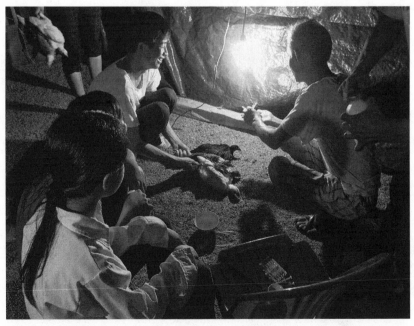

FIG. 4. Newcastle vaccination on Thủy and Trí's semi-commercial chicken farm in Bắc Giang province. Trí's cousin, Mịnh, presents the birds to Ông Đức for inoculation while Trí prepares the solution and Thủy gathers more birds. Thủy and Trí's daughter and neighbor look on, ready to help with the solution as needed. Photo by author.

coordinated effort made possible by Trí's direction, his father's experience, and the efficient help of family and neighbors. However, the service was not free, and I soon realized why Mịnh was so jovial upon his arrival. After we exited the coop, Thủy sent Qui back to the house to pick up the rice porridge she prepared earlier in the day, and Trí ventured into his father's place where he had stored a case of Hanoi beer to share (a treat for villagers accustomed to home-brewed rice wine). We sat outside into the night, joking and drinking as more neighbors passed in and out of the courtyard. Several weeks later I would find myself at Mịnh's house with Trí, reciprocating the labor by vaccinating Mịnh's flock for Newcastle, and then enjoying some popsicles and beer.

The family-based labor relations in place for Newcastle virus did not translate to H5N1. Farmers like Trí transport poultry products across district lines, which means they must have a certificate that says their birds have been vaccinated against bird flu. To obtain this certificate, Trí, Thủy and Ông Đức were forced to seek out the assistance of a state-certified vet. They did so begrudgingly. Like many of the farmers I met, Trí complained that Duy, their district veterinarian, had little sense of the practical realities (kinh nghiệm thực tế) of poultry production. He also stated that state veterinarians were corrupt. One night I told Trí and Thủy that a state-employed veterinarian in a neighboring district was about to retire and only worked sporadically in her capacity as a veterinarian. Thủy huffed, "It's not because she's about to retire, it's because she's a state employee . . . they have no idea what goes on with the farmers . . . Ông Duy [the People's Committee vet in their district] is the same way! We know better about what medicines to give, and we go and buy them ourselves. They don't give us any help with farming." Trí agreed:

> The state agents don't ever come to see us or help us. . . . I don't want to speak ill of people, but the People's Committee is really corrupt. They keep all the resources for themselves and don't interact with farmers. They even take things that the government sets aside for the people and resell them. Ông Duy does that. The government provides free bird flu vaccines to the people, but he doesn't give it to us. He resells it instead. He's a certified sales agent, you know. All of the state vets have their own shops and sell the stuff from the government to make their own profit.[3]

Thủy and Trí took issue with what they saw as an unjust distribution of rights and resources in vaccination strategies. Not only did they see state vets as ignorant about farmers' situations and animal health in general, in Vietnam's unregulated and increasingly privatized health sector, state vets could easily fashion themselves as private vets, and in doing so seek profits that stripped farmers of their entitlements to state subsidized, "public" health therapies. Growing up in the shadows of a socialized health care system, and amid a nationalist discourse that couches government policies in the interests of the people, it was not surprising that Trí and Thủy were angry that state services eluded them—that is, when they thought vaccines were being appropriated by the very people responsible for their public provision. As one farmer told me rather poetically, "*Kiểm soát là kiếm tiền,*" to control [bird flu] is to make money.

No matter how much they resented this form of governance, Thủy and Trí were required to seek state veterinary services for HPAI vaccination. A few months after my arrival in Placid Pond, their flock was due for inoculation. The couple elected to enlist the services of a paravet to complete the job. Even though they had just a few weeks of training at most, Thủy and Trí drew on their services because paravets were known to be more readily available than full-time vets (largely because they were younger and engaged in fewer income-generating activities). I knew that the HPAI vaccination would proceed differently than other animal inoculations when, a few minutes before the paravet's arrival, Trí's aunt came to Ông Đức's house clutching several rather skinny chickens. The hens were part of Trí and Thủy's flock, but were kept at her house for lack of space. These were "spent hens" past their laying prime. Thủy joined Trí's aunt and mother as they worked to slaughter the chickens before the arrival of the veterinarian. "Clean them up well, niece," Trí's aunt instructed. "Too bad they're so skinny." Though they were not officially required to pay for the HPAI vaccine, the family was expected to provide some form of compensation for the veterinarian's time, and these birds, though skinny, would suffice.

By the time the paravet arrived, Thủy had sequestered the flock behind a tarp and hung a lantern above a plastic chair in the corner of the coop. Trí invited the young man to sit down on a chair so that he and Ông Đức could present the animals to him, again in groups of three. I had never seen an inoculation carried out from this position: Trí's family squatted when they probed the birds, and the state vets I worked with vaccinated from a standing position. Though he lacked a pristine white lab coat, the paravet used the same pistol-like syringes employed by Mai and her team (those that connected directly to the bottle of vaccine and administered pre-measured amounts of solution). The device allowed him to work quickly, and though he was the only one injecting he finished the job in less time than it took for the whole family to carry out the Newcastle inoculation. Throughout the process, Trí was even tenser than when vaccinating on his own. Like Ông Cường observing how I injected his ducks, Trí scrutinized the man's work, but made an effort not to stare or offer suggestions. It was only after they sent the paravet home with the chickens (he tersely refused the family's offer of beer), that Trí commented on his technique, noting that how quickly he worked. Ông Đức tried to reassure him. "Yeah, those guys are always in a hurry to finish. But he did an O.K. job." Addled and anxious to talk more about the inoculation, Trí explained to me that one had to watch paravets because they were minimally trained young people looking to make some easy income. He said that Ông Đức would do just as good a job, but state-certified veterinarians had a monopoly on bird flu vaccines as well as the inoculation certifications necessary for poultry trade.[4]

I would add that Trí's careful observation of the paravet also stemmed from the fact that his presence disrupted the social networks and agreements—forms of life—that Trí generally drew on for poultry care. Whenever I asked whom the local veterinary experts were, farmers would more often than not point to a practicing chicken producer in the village rather than a public, paravet, or private vet. For example, though he did not work professionally as a vet, Trí's uncle Lơ studied veterinary medicine for several years and often fielded phone calls and visits from farmers with questions about unusual livestock symptoms. When I asked farmers why they sought out Lơ, I found that he derived his authority from formal education as well as years of practical experience raising chickens. Trí was particularly reliant on Lơ because of their familial relationship. Lơ lived just twenty meters away from Trí, frequently consulted with Trí and his father on chicken medication and feeding regimes, and even provided some of the initial funds needed to send Thủy to Taiwan to work as an au pair. These familial and financial ties meant that Lơ was invested in the well-being of Trí and his animals, and that he was intimately involved in all manner of animal care. I remember clearly one morning when I awoke to terrifying, unidentifiable screeching, only to run out to the patio and witness Lơ neutering Thủy and Trí's fully alert family dog with a dull razor blade pinched between two fingers. The pup had recently been on a few tears in the village and had Thủy at her wits' end. Lơ, it seemed, had located the source of the problem in the poor beast's gonads. Their uncle's consultation on this and other animal health issues suggests that it was not necessarily the veterinary activities that farmers found objectionable, but rather the idea that a state agent rather than their own relatives should carry them out.

When I asked what the vet was going to do with all the chickens, Trí's aunt replied that he would give them to his relatives. "Lucky them," she noted with sarcasm. Unlike the jovial atmosphere following the Newcastle vaccination, everyone was reticent, somewhat sour, that evening. It was clear that the family was not friendly with the paravet, and I had not seen him in the village before or after the vaccination. Thủy was particularly upset. She had griped and moaned while slaughtering the chickens, "Five chickens for five minutes!" she muttered, rousing a cackle from her aunt and mother-in-law. Ông Đức liked to say that Thủy was born in the sign of the dragon and could be *khó tính*, difficult, or hard-hearted. Especially when it came to financial matters, she could sometimes get very unpleasant. But I think that Thủy was upset at more than the cost of inoculation. Like Trí, she was reacting to the fact that the paravet's presence generated new exchange relations on the family farm. To be sure, these relations placed financial responsibilities on the family's shoulders, but they also brought unfamiliar persons with less than enviable expertise into biological contact with the family flock.

Thủy was particularly concerned about how vet-administered inoculation would affect the productivity of the birds, since hens have been known to lay fewer eggs in the aftermath of bird flu vaccination. Vietnamese poultry have historically been more valued for their egg rather than meat production (Smith and Daniel 2000, 33), and Thủy had worked out her own manner of handling the hens during inoculation. She would clutch their legs very close to the ground, far away from their stomachs and reproductive organs. And after the birds had been probed and swept aside, Thủy would position herself in between them and the overhead lamp in an attempt to shield their eyes and avoid further shock. The paravet's presence, however, alienated Thủy and her female relatives from work of enumerating immunity. Though they figured centrally in the Newcastle vaccination, during the bird flu inoculation female family members were relegated to the back of the house to slaughter chickens, and wait. This was a stark reversal of roles, since in daily practice it was Thủy and her mother-in-law, Bà An, who were largely responsible for caring for the hens (Trí dealt with traders and drove the eggs to neighboring markets, and Ông Đức ran the household hatchery). The paravet thus upset the gendered, collaborative kinship relations that structured poultry care, relations that traditionally followed the maxim, *nhất thân, nhì quên*, "first family, then familiar."[5]

Conclusion

Whether for poultry or people, vaccines raise a host of difficult questions about how to distribute life-saving devices in pandemic contexts. I have shown here how these questions come to the fore in the everyday work of poultry vaccination, or, more specifically, in the exchanges between state vets, farmers, and poultry. As the arm of the state responsible for carrying out inoculations in farming communities, vets like Mai have been credited with their central role in national efforts to enumerate immunity in avian and human populations. And indeed, by some estimates, Mai and her colleagues have had significant success. Since the campaign began, no poultry or human outbreaks have been traced to fully vaccinated flocks (Peyre et al. 2011).[6] Such measurable outcomes align well with what Melissa Pashigian (2012) argues is an increasingly assessment-oriented health arena in Vietnam, in which counting and enumeration serve as justification for novel and controversial medical interventions. Like the IVF treatments Pashigian documents, H5N1 poultry vaccines were newcomers to Vietnam, and as such health officials and citizens relied on counting practices as metrics for success. Processes of enumerating immunity have engendered a situation in which the ostensibly temporary "first phase" vaccination measure has become a protracted technical solution to the problem of defending human lives against animal viruses.

But even though the vaccine experiment endures in rural communities, its initial target and objectives have become skewed, and its methods and outcomes have changed. In principle, mass vaccination relies on sustained poultry inoculations as part of a future-oriented effort to preempt avian infection and the possibility of spillover that could generate a human-to-human flu strain. In practice, however, many farmers frequently waited for poultry outbreaks to occur before seeking vaccination, and Mai's immunization activities did less to anticipate the human pandemic than they did to respond to ongoing poultry infections. For this and other reasons, the vaccine solution to the pandemic problem has given some health strategists pause. As the senior epidemiologist referenced above had it, "The policy is not working," and needs to be replaced with more sustainable disease-control measures that target not just the virus, but also the ecological and economic conditions that give rise to infectious agents.

My observations of the ways that vaccines circulated in farming communities revealed still other uncertainties. By anticipating an emerging but not yet present human pandemic event, vaccine experiments did not fully address the current situation in which H5N1 had become endemic to domestic poultry, decimating avian populations and farmers livelihoods. Poultry health and economic concerns were at the forefront of farmers' minds when they considered vaccination, and because vaccine strategies elided those concerns, their appeal diminished. Vaccine strategies also occluded more pressing pathogenic threats. By honing in on potentially pandemic H5N1 viruses, vaccination policies overlooked the critical role that other pathogens play in Vietnam's livestock economies. The fact that farmers were more concerned about poultry health than human health, more preoccupied with pigs than ducks, and more afraid of Newcastle than bird flu, indicates that there are multiple valuations of life forms, and multiple estimations of risk in the economies where HPAI surfaces. Vets weighed these diverse concerns as they made decisions about how to incorporate HPAI vaccines into their other disease-control activities.

Vets' vaccination decisions also reflected the limited resources they had on hand at any given time, and their creative attempts to make do in Vietnam's transitioning health system. Vaccine supplies were a constant preoccupation among state vets. They circulated within a chronically underfunded and under-resourced public animal health sector, one that has been losing traction in light of the ongoing privatization of human and animal health services. Importantly, privatization posed both risks and opportunities for state vets. Even though failure to achieve immunity in their jurisdictions put vets at risk for financial penalty and farmers' scorn, the heterogeneous pool of veterinary actors emerging in Vietnam provided avenues for generating income and other benefits from private entrepreneurial activities. The vets I describe here all transited between public and private animal health sectors to pursue their individual livelihood strategies. This was risky business, though, because the fact that state veterinarians moonlighted in the private sector raised questions about whose rights and interests were actually driving the distribution of "public" health therapies. And so although many global health strategists have lauded the Vietnamese government for successfully bringing H5N1 governance into line with established state structures, for many, the ways in which vaccines changed hands between the state and citizens fell short.

Of course, farmers were not only concerned about the possibility that state vets were appropriating public vaccine supplies. They also worried about whether state vaccines and state vaccinators could properly safeguard poultry. Poultry health was the primary concern for many farmers I met in Bắc Giang and Đồng Tháp, most of who did not buy into public discourses about human flu risks. In contrast to One Health rhetoric, farmers did not take interspecies zoonotic transmission as given, and instead viewed mundane corporeal exchanges between species as productive, even immunizing, not dangerous. In Vietnam, H5N1 is endemic to poultry and very rare in humans, and the idea that humans could be put at risk by poultry does not sit well with a historical and cultural tradition that has long celebrated intimate, fleshy relations between species. Marianne Lien puts it nicely when she suggests that whether a domesticated animal is a vector or a victim depends on one's positioning (2015, 30). And so, within the context of unanticipated human outbreaks, farmers shifted the target and objective of vaccination away from human immunity toward poultry immunity, and in doing so redefined the exchange relations through which vaccination should proceed. Ông Đức, Thủy, and Trí preferred to pursue immunity through established kin relationships in which the care of poultry was as important as the control of viruses. Although vets by and large respected these preferences, laboring under a regime of H5N1 governance meant that they had to insert themselves into the daily work of vaccination. And inasmuch as the public provision of bird flu vaccines failed to honor long-standing forms of animal care that brought farmers and fowl into fleshy contact, they aroused mistrust and even anger among farmers who begrudged the transient and largely unaccountable work of state agents.

Taken together, these tales of vaccination signal the myriad problems involved with singling out viruses as the target of a "quick fix" One Health experiment, as well as the myriad problems involved with singling out state veterinarians as the primary implementers of flu governance. Like the H5N1 virus itself, vets stand at the crossroads of public health and poultry business, and they were tasked with balancing the multiple risks, interests, and responsibilities therein. That they struggled to achieve this balance was no fault of their own, but rather was a symptom of a larger disjuncture in One Health agendas to incorporate human and animal health without fully considering the political ecologies, livestock economies, and social relations—forms of life—in which life forms meet. The irony of vaccine experiments is that they proceeded from an assumption that the integration of human and nonhuman animal health is a new phenomenon in rural Vietnam, when in fact poultry farmers have long recognized their shared vulnerabilities with other species, and addressed them by engaging in forms of care that target humans, livestock, and livelihoods *together*. Though they contrasted with One Health strategies, farmers' approaches to livestock care revealed themselves to be more diverse, more attuned to interspecies entanglements, and more sensitive to changing local environments and economies, than the quick fix promised by vaccines.

3

Commerce and Containment

Closing time approaches at Bến Thành market in the heart of Ho Chi Minh City's commercial district. Near the Eastern Gate, tourists stow away their lacquer and silks as they prepare to haggle for a ride back to their hotels. Housewives walk briskly to their motorbikes and bicycles, on whose handlebars they dangle baggies filled with makings for their evening meals. At the opposite end, past the teas and pickled vegetables, beyond the rice noodle and fresh juice vendors, lies the Western Gate. The ground here is saturated by running water, which carries a mix of debris and blood away from the stalls and out to the street. Flies scatter and reassemble around meat in motion as pork vendors deftly stack raw flesh into bamboo baskets, readying it for the journey home. Catfish struggle against the grasping hands that would remove them from their plastic pools, and street dogs dodge swinging broomsticks in their quest for errant scraps. At the end of this line of merchants, in a corner brightened by fluorescent light, Nhuẩn observes the activity from his position behind a freezer. His impassive face is illuminated by a sign overhead promising, "Fresh and Processed Poultry, Clean and Safe." He assures me, "The city is safe. We don't worry about bird flu here. The problem is over there, in the countryside, where they still eat unprocessed chicken."

I had ventured into Bến Thành market in search of the chicken retailers I had become accustomed to in Ho Chi Minh City in 2003: those selling fowl at every stage of the life cycle. At that time, if you were in the market for a live chicken, *gà sống* could be found under domes of woven bamboo—their vitality on display as a sign of good health and flavor. An extra fee would have your bird butchered on site; otherwise you could slaughter it at home. If you were in a hurry, prepared varieties were readily available; simply look up and choose from the bodies hanging overhead. Or then again, if an entire bird fell out of range of your pocketbook or appetite, you might consider a processed chicken, whose partible bits were available for inspection and purchase. But this was several years after outbreaks of H5N1 began decimating millions of birds and killing citizens with equal impunity. Ample time, that is, to rearrange the face and flesh of Vietnam's urban poultry markets.

Since outbreaks of SARS and bird flu were first traced to live animal markets in Asian metropolises, these spaces of multispecies exchange have become critical sites of health intervention. Bến Thành market bore the mark of these interventions. It had taken me over thirty minutes to even find Nhuẩn, who seemed to be one of only a small handful of poultry vendors in a market once brimming with chicken. Once I found him, the contrast between Nhuẩn and his flesh-flinging counterparts was striking. While his neighbors continued to work closely with raw pork and live fish, Nhuẩn followed orders from Ho Chi Minh City authorities to sell ducks and chickens only after they had been raised, processed, and packaged by an industrial-integrated, commercial farm.[1] In this lively market, people-poultry-pathogen entanglements were limited by layers of procedural and material containment: layers that not only rendered poultry into commodities, but also structured the habits, practices, and ideas of producers, vendors, and consumers.

Vietnam's market restrictions marked a transition away from targeted, quick-fix experiments like vaccinations, toward farther-reaching, "sustainable" experiments centered on restructuring domestic poultry production. In their broadest sense, market restrictions placed limits on how poultry could be produced, processed, and sold to urban consumers. These limits were put in place for two reasons: to reduce the risk of HPAI outbreaks, and to test whether Vietnam could feasibly transition to industrially integrated commercial poultry production, a system in which all aspects of production and marketing are owned and regulated by a single company. Market restrictions were experimental; there was no guarantee that either of these goals would be achieved. For one thing, consumer preference for local, homegrown poultry suggested that there might not actually be a demand for industrially produced commercial varieties in Vietnam. For another, the links between industrial production and biological safety remain unclear (Davis 2005), and when market restrictions were implemented there was no definitive evidence demonstrating that poultry produced in these systems was less vulnerable to HPAI. In the context of such uncertainties, market restrictions were piloted in Vietnamese cities as experiments that would allow policy makers to collect evidence on whether a consumer base could be established for industrially produced commercial poultry, and whether increased sales of this kind of meat could be linked to outbreak reductions.

If successful, market restriction experiments would go a long way toward reaching the government's goal of transforming the composition of the national livestock sector—a goal with economic as well as sociocultural implications. The industrialization of Vietnam's poultry would push millions of local poultry varieties and their small-scale producers out of Vietnam's expanding urban markets, and prohibit transactions that have long provided much needed income for the rural poor. In addition to these economic effects, market restrictions would also exacerbate existing symbolic divisions between inside and outside, country and city in Vietnam. For urban dwellers like Nhuẩn, this experiment was turning a once idealized Vietnamese countryside into a health hazard, a place of bad bugs and bad behavior. In market restrictions, then, epidemiological evaluations were tangled up with economic and moral ones.

I now turn to analyze bird flu governance beyond the farm and down the commodity chain, by examining market restrictions in and around Hanoi and Ho Chi Minh City. In contrast to biosecurity and vaccination experiments, which modify poultry biologies and on the farm ecologies, market restrictions regulate all of the serial transactions that bring poultry from farm to market. I begin by describing how market restrictions instilled measures to contain the activities and movements of Vietnamese poultry and producers. I then recount the experiences of farmers who responded differently to such restrictions. I show that while some farmers complied with containment measures to tap into new commodity chains, others inventively moved through space to maintain control over the products of their labor, and to access a range of livestock markets. In the midst of market restrictions, poultry followed both sanctioned and unsanctioned pathways to and from the city; and as they moved through space they engaged in a variety of exchange relationships with humans—each of which entailed culturally and historically specific obligations, dependencies, and proprietary arrangements. Taken together, I suggest that the varied outcomes of market restriction experiments reflect an ongoing struggle between the Vietnamese state and citizens over the value of different livestock commodities, and the future of different livelihood strategies.

By most counts, poultry production systems in Vietnam have failed to keep up with rising demand, particularly in urban centers. The integrated commercial systems common to industrial societies in the Global North, in which one company controls all stages in poultry production, have grown slowly in Vietnam, and small and medium-scale systems continue to dominate the country's poultry sector (Hong Hanh, Burgos, and Roland-Holst 2007, 10).[2]

In these latter systems, poultry have much more freedom of movement and tend to change hands across a variety of hatchers, growers, slaughterers, processors, transporters, and vendors as they transit to city markets. But freedom and mobility pose problems for bird flu governance, and health experts argued that such unregulated exchanges expose poultry to different hosts and pathogens, thereby increasing risks for all manner of infection. As one transnational study summarizes:

> Small and medium scale commercial production has been able to expand very fast to meet demand gaps in newly growing economies such as Vietnam, and in the areas immediately surrounding many large cities of the developing world. . . . However, in the countries where supply has grown fastest, it has not been matched by an expansion of safety and quality regulation in livestock food chains (Mcleod, Thieme, and Mack 2009, 192).

The persistence of unregulated poultry commodity chains in Vietnam and elsewhere has ignited concerns among health strategists about how to govern poultry traffic between country and city.[3] Enter market restrictions. In Vietnam, market restrictions began by prohibiting poultry production in large cities and limiting the sale and slaughter of live birds in urban areas. Restrictions also sought to control the movements of rural poultry producers by placing quarantines on inter-district and interprovincial trade, which reduced opportunities for smallholding poultry producers to access city markets on their own or via traders. As H5N1 outbreaks continued, market restrictions piloted new ways to further restrict this access—namely, by regulating the kinds and quality of poultry varieties available to urban consumers. Particularly in Ho Chi Minh City, market restrictions have limited poultry sales to industrially integrated commercial varieties—those "clean and safe" birds peddled by vendors like Nhuẫn.

Taken together, market restrictions targeted what flu planners term "poultry value chains," or the range of activities that bring a poultry product (live animal, meat, eggs) to consumers. Value chain interventions comprised measures to create "value-added products" by controlling the activities of producers, processors, transporters, retailers, and consumers (Rota and Sperandini 2010, 1). The NSCAI's Green Book delineated several plans for regulating these activities:

> Poultry production in large cities (such as Ho Chi Minh City and Hanoi) should be discouraged and eventually prohibited. Slaughterhouses should be located away from residential areas to minimize public health risks and environmental nuisance. The marketing of poultry will be regulated, and it is expected that industrialization would lead to increased sales of processed

product, especially in urban areas (National Steering Committee on Human and Avian Influenza 2006c, vii).[4]

This policy statement shows how market restrictions brought public health and commercial interests into productive relation. According to this future-oriented statement, experimental modifications to the poultry value chain not only mitigate health risks; they also provide a regulatory framework for testing consumer demand for commercial meat.

Industrializing Organisms, Compromising Lives

The industrial-integrated commercial poultry (*gia cầm công nghiệp*) piloted in urban markets differ considerably from poultry raised on small and medium farms in Vietnam. First, in terms of the animals themselves, commercial breeds feature growth and productivity rates that far outstrip the native and hybrid varieties common to smaller operations. Industrial-integrated commercial meat tends to be drier, softer, and less sinewy than the meat traditionally favored by Vietnamese consumers. As one FAO advisor told me over a bowl of phở gà (chicken noodle soup), "It's not like this stringy meat that gets stuck between your teeth." Second, in terms of production, commercial poultry exists in large-scale industrial holdings where thousands of birds cohabitate in climate controlled, enclosed shelters, eating the same feed and engaging in the same limited, movements meant to fatten flesh in the fastest manner possible. Third, while poultry is traditionally bought live and slaughtered at home or at the point of sale, industrial-integrated fowl are slaughtered and processed in-house according to company standards, and reach the consumer as a prepackaged, branded product.

In further contrast to small- and medium-scale operations, industrial-integrated commercial poultry production also requires substantial financial investments (in breeding and feeding technologies, in production and processing infrastructures, and in marketing methods). Both central and local government agencies have thus offered credit with preferential interest rates to encourage farmers to experiment with industrializing their holdings. Mass organizations and local-level People's Committee offices also provided farmers with technical training in breeding techniques, animal health inputs, and commercial marketing strategies. In addition to this governmental support, multinational bird flu strategists and major commercial poultry producers have helped finance Vietnam's industrialization process. Commercial companies such as Thailand's CP (Charoen Popkhand) Foods, Singaporean-based JAPFA, and Vietnam's own 99 Poultry have continued to gain a stronger foothold in the poultry sector by establishing contracts with farmers who adhere to industry standards and expand their market base.

These initiatives formed part of a longer-term ten-year HPAI strategy developed by the Ministry of Agriculture and Rural Development (MARD). MARD hoped to see industrialized and semi-industrialized poultry farms account for 80 percent of domestic poultry production by 2015, with scattered small-scale household farms making up the rest. Though it did not reach its target, Vietnamese poultry production has changed significantly since market restrictions began to take effect. According to a comprehensive economic assessment of bird flu policies, market restrictions have "reduced the scope for [small scale, semi-commercial] producers to access the high-end market for poultry and generally the market for any poultry in the large urban centers like Hanoi and HCMC; relegating them to being suppliers to small retail vendors in district and provincial markets" (Agrifood Consulting International 2007, 260). Large numbers of small-scale farmers left the industry in the first year after restrictions took effect, including 20 percent of semi-commercial and household producers (Pham and Roland-Holst 2007). In fact, if implemented thoroughly, restructuring would push over eight million households out of smallholding and semi-commercial poultry production (Vu 2009).

Avian flu policy statements naturalize the losses to small-scale farmers. The Ministry of Agriculture and Rural Development predicted early on that a "large number" of households that had produced poultry on a small scale "shall change to other, more profitable jobs" such as wage laborers in large-scale slaughtering and processing enterprises (National Steering Committee on Human and Avian Influenza 2006b, 27). Similarly, the Green Book states that household poultry production "in the longer term is likely to erode naturally in densely populated areas as other enterprises take the place of poultry rearing" (National Steering Committee on Human and Avian Influenza 2006c, vii). Multinational bird flu strategists agreed. The aforementioned economic assessment concludes, "In essence, while traders were hit hard during the actual outbreaks and many left the industry, those that remained or reentered found a more lucrative market for their products" (Agrifood Consulting International 2007, 238). Market restrictions thus took on a kind of inevitability in official rhetoric, which maintained an optimistic outlook on losses to smallholders by highlighting producers who increased their level of industrialization and confined their market activities to commercial trade networks. According to this story, such entrepreneurial farmers generated higher profits from increased consumer demand for certified, biosafe poultry.

But there is another, less frequently told story about market restrictions, which involves not only their economic, but also their social and biological consequences. These consequences stemmed from the ways in which market restrictions pressured farmers to alter their land use practices and their exchange relations with poultry. As part of its long-term HPAI strategy, the Vietnamese government has been zoning different types of land for large-scale production and processing, and industrial operations have taken over large swaths of land in order to house animals in facilities far removed from households. Emerging land tenure systems have required farmers with industrial, commercial aspirations to move away from natal households and villages. Such moves, however, call for capital, and some policy analysts suggested that

> land use and land tenure systems that promote safe and environmentally friendly poultry production may involve zoning of production and processing. If zoning regulations are put into place to force the sector to restructure, small firms will be at a disadvantage in competing for land on which to site their production units and markets (Mcleod, Thieme, and Mack 2009, 197).

I will describe how land use changes disadvantage small farmers below. Here I want to note that statements like this frame poultry sector restructuring in a metric of market driven competition, and rely on the notion that industrialization will be propelled by rising consumer demand for commercial poultry in urban areas. In 2005, economists began conducting research to ascertain urban consumer preferences with regard to live or processed poultry, as well as their willingness to source commercial meat from supermarkets in lieu of buying live animals at wet markets. On the whole they found limited support for commercial products. For instance, even though southern city dwellers were more receptive to processed, certified poultry varieties than their northern counterparts at the onset of outbreaks, studies conducted a few years after H5N1 became endemic indicated that southerners were turning back to local, non-commercial brands (Ifft et al. 2010).

Northerners, too, have continued to demand local chicken. This is especially true during the Tết Lunar New Year holiday, by far the most important, and, in terms of H5N1, dangerous holiday in the country. Government officials, multinational experts, and citizens alike had all come to expect H5N1 outbreaks to increase across the country around Tết, especially in urban areas like Hanoi and Ho Chi Minh City. Health experts cited two primary reasons for heightened pestilence. First, that Tết falls in the winter months when flus, colds, and other illnesses are on the rise. This is a time when people and poultry alike must beware of *gió bắc*: northern winds that blow into households and bodies, causing chills and general malaise. Tết season, in other words, is flu season. Second, as one FAO consultant put it to me, "There's just a helluva lot more chicken in the country during the New Year," as families prepare chickens for ancestral altars, and to feast on with relatives and friends.

In an effort to stem holiday outbreaks, bird flu strategists discouraged city-bound traffic in live animals. Animal health officials worked with local authorities to implement poultry checks at district and provincial borders. City veterinarians increased their market visits, prevailing upon vendors for vaccine certificates and documents that delineated the source of their fowl. Those occupying the edges of city markets, the street hawkers so ubiquitous in Hanoi, faced fines if found with live chicken. All of this against the background noise of public health messages that issued a slew of warnings in state-run newspapers, on television shows, and over neighborhood loudspeakers: don't buy live poultry; purchase safe and processed varieties in your local supermarket or from certified vendors; look for vaccination certification; and never, under any circumstances, buy from unknown sources.

Still, in spite of all of the anticipation and preparation, bird flu outbreaks have continually increased in Ho Chi Minh City and Hanoi around the New Year, and these outbreaks are often traced to flocks that should have never arrived in the cities in the first place. How has this happened? To answer this question, I traveled a few dozen kilometers from Hanoi's city center to Hà Vĩ market, Vietnam's largest poultry wholesaler.[5]

At daybreak I navigated my rented Honda motorbike through Hanoi's city center, traveling on a dyke road flanked by a mosaic depicting vibrant scenes from Vietnamese history (a unique beautification project in a city often criticized for losing its charm to overdevelopment). Crossing Long Biên Bridge over the Red River was slow going. Aggressive truck drivers vied for space against hundreds of motorbikes like my own, while overburdened buses struggled to move people and their wares out of the city. From the opposite direction came a comparable number of commuters weighed down by commodities destined for city markets. Hanoi's notorious motorbikes of burden hauled everything from plastic bins to air conditioners to rebar wires to live animals. Caged puppies made their way to Hanoi's infamous dog meat stalls, where they would be sacrificed to fill the bellies of men in search of heat-generating canine flesh (said to confer immunity in the winter). Pigs were hogtied to motorbikes on their way to a similar fate. Chickens, too, were headed to the city center. Handfuls of birds sat upright in bicycle baskets while others swung suspended from handlebars. Motorbikes could carry more, and I spotted several hundred dangling from the backs and front of Hondas, while still more birds stood stationed in between drivers' legs.

I knew from policy papers, national media reports, and prior interviews that the majority of these cyclists and motorbike drivers would be unable to provide any kind of certification for the birds; that is, whether they were vaccinated for H5N1 or from what producer they came. I also knew that many of these traders had traveled up to hundreds of kilometers to reach Hanoi's city markets where they could sell eggs, chicks, and full-grown fowl at a higher price than in their villages. These idiosyncrasies occupied my mind as the highway opened up. As I increased my distance from Hanoi, bicycles, motorbikes, and pedestrians were replaced by scores of trucks making their way to the city center from which I had come. I turned down a long dirt path from which these vehicles appeared and came upon what looked like a normal row of pastel-colored two- and three-story houses. But in their entryways and reception areas I did not glimpse the usual tea services or storefront operations; instead I only saw chickens and ducks, hundreds and thousands of chickens and ducks. The houses seemed to be hemorrhaging birds. Birds of different breeds, brands, colors, and ages occupied every conveyance imaginable: bamboo cages, plastic crates, rice sacks, plastic bags. And trucks kept pulling in; already teeming with birds they generated a cloud of dust and feathers in their wake. Men jumped out and started packing in thousands more, moving from one vendor to another seemingly without communication or negotiation, the only sound the steady squawk of startled fowl.

A plump vendor in her twenties waved me over as I dismounted my motorbike. Keen to talk, Yến invited me to pass the day with her under a tarpaulin cover that shielded us from a steady winter drizzle. As we casually surveyed the market activity, Yến explained that she did not deal with the large transporters moving in and out of the market. She sourced her birds from three farms in neighboring provinces and brought them by motorbike to Ha Vĩ in order to sell to smaller operations—namely, restaurateurs buying the evening's meat, or traders bringing modest batches to local markets. Those picking up fewer animals did a bit more shopping around, she said, and we waited patiently for them to circle back to us after assessing the other birds on offer.

Digging at her cuticle beds, Yến observed, "You picked a slow day, little sister. Tomorrow is when it gets busy here."

"This is a slow day?" I asked, surprised. "Is it because everyone's supposed to shop at the supermarkets?"

"Oh stop it (*thôi*). Saturday is busier is all. Nobody likes supermarket chicken, and of course we can't eat it during Tết. For Tết it has to be local (our) chicken (*gà ta*). And they're always better live. . . . Otherwise, how can you tell if they're healthy?"

This was a conversation I had had many, many times before, and one that corroborated my observations of poultry consumption in Hanoi and Ho Chi Minh City. Every visit I had ever made to the supermarkets, where industrially integrated commercial poultry is sold in freezers, felt eerily lonely. Situated in upscale malls or near high-rise apartment complexes catering to foreign diplomats, these stores seemed to specialize in imported items: Haribo gummy candies from Germany, Oreo cookies from the United States, Présidénte butter from France. The clientele was made up of expatriates or well-to-do Vietnamese who, even though they could afford the items, seemed to be visiting the supermarket as a social outing. Even those Vietnamese working in the field of bird flu control refrained from buying supermarket poultry, and some openly anticipated visits to the countryside where the birds are still considered healthier.

In addition to wrongly hypothesizing a demand for industrial poultry, market restrictions also acted on incomplete scientific data about the relationship between industrial production and virus control. Rooted in modernization schemes started in revolutionary era, poultry-sector restructuring has gained new urgency with the onset of H5N1 outbreaks, as policy makers and health strategists link industrial production methods to increased biosecurity. But there are those who question the assumed connection between industrialization and disease control, and criticize its effects on smallholding rural producers. According to a study conducted by the FAO's Pro-Poor Livestock Policy Initiative

> these scale biases in livestock development policy reinforce the processes of structural change in the sector and sharpen the disadvantages of poor rural smallholders. In large part because of HPAI induced poultry mortalities and the assumption that smallholder systems have higher disease risk levels. . . . However, scientifically it has not yet been clearly established that larger and concentrated poultry production systems are inherently safer than small, decentralized ones (Hong Hanh, Burgos, and Roland-Holst 2007, 10).

Going further, a 2009 study by the same research group argues that although it is often assumed that "confined" food animal production reduces the risk of zoonotic diseases, evidence suggests that industrial-integrated systems may actually *increase* both animal and public health risks. "Although not typically recognized as such, industrial food animal production generates unique ecosystems—environments that may facilitate the evolution of zoonotic pathogens and their transmission to human populations" (Leibler et al. 2009, 1).[6]

My own conversations with animal health experts supported these findings. Throughout my research, there was a growing suspicion among animal health experts that large-scale poultry farms were the ones in need of governance, and that the NSCAI's focus on small- and medium-scale farms might have been misinformed. One transnational veterinary advisor told me, "There is an abundance of expert opinion with little scientific research." Another wrote in an email:

> The organizations you will work with/observe . . . started by following their normal target group, poor farmers. The risks so far as we can tell are much more loaded into the commercial sector. There has been a gradual realization that scavenging backyard producers may not be most at risk. Personally I feel small farmers are victims of a misjudgment by the international community and veterinary services, the evidence was simply not there when an intuitive decision was required. . . . Development agencies followed their biases in assuming that poor, small-scale farmers would be most affected, most vulnerable (HPAI technical advisor, November 24, 2008).

There is also anecdotal evidence indicating that what makes poor farmers most vulnerable are not small-scale production systems, but rather poultry sector restructuring policies. News accounts raised questions about the effects of industrial-integration on rural farmers. While many stories celebrated entrepreneurial farmers who adopted industrial modes of production, more critical accounts of this process appeared on Vietnam's state-controlled television stations VTV News and periodicals such as *Thành Niên* and *Tuổi Trẻ*. These alternative narratives featured farmers, often with tears in their eyes, who found themselves no longer able to sell their flocks at key markets.

And yet, in spite of lingering questions about the scientific validity of industrial farming for disease control, the questionable consumer demand for industrially produced poultry, and the effects of value chain modifications on poor rural farmers, market restrictions continue apace in Vietnam. The persistence of these experiments indicates that market restrictions have been driven by more than epidemiological, or even economic, considerations. I want to suggest that the market restrictions reflect ambivalent ideas about the place of rural landscapes, farmers, and fowl in Vietnam's commercializing economy. Anthropologist Philip Taylor explains:

> To this day, planners entertain high modernist ambitions for the socialist industrialization of the countryside. Billboards with images of tractors plowing fields, electricity pylons spanning the countryside, factories belching smoke, and industrial workers in overalls and hard hats are situated in the middle of rice fields throughout the country, signaling the desire of Vietnam's leaders that their overwhelmingly agricultural nation leap into full-fledged modernity (Taylor 2007, 12).

Discourses like this draw on a long-standing, ideological separation of city and country in Vietnam. This separation, and the higher value afforded to

cities, have animated governing systems that target rural areas as sites of social and political engineering and experimentation. Such discourses have also
fueled concerns about how to securitize city boundaries in light of HPAI outbreaks, and driven efforts to keep "undeveloped," "polluted," rural products
out of urban environments.

Of course, in Vietnam, as elsewhere, rural and urban categories do not
coincide with bounded, material spaces, but rather are conceptual categories
that provide models for social organization.[7] The idealized duality (Harms
2011, 2) that holds city and country apart in Vietnam is especially difficult
to maintain in a national context where boundaries between country and
city are increasingly fluid. Erik Harms (2011) carefully illustrates this fact by
showing how labor and commodity chains link rural and urban spaces and
promote, even demand, social, material, and discursive exchanges between
country and city. Against this background, market restrictions reflect ambivalence about forms of life that increasingly promote the mobility of "rural"
people and poultry in Vietnam, thereby permitting them to penetrate city
boundaries with "outside" and potentially dangerous pathogens. Farmers
played with this ambivalence, taking their own view on what counts as inside
and outside, city and country. Many farmers chose not to take restrictions
that circumscribed their access to urban markets at face value, and instead
maneuvered within poultry value chains in ways that accorded with their
own livelihood traditions and entrepreneurial ambitions. In what follows, I
take a granular view of these maneuvers.

Thủy and Trí

With its high population densities and limited land, the Red River Delta has
become home to high-volume household chicken farms that the NSCAI is
trying to eradicate, namely by encouraging producers to move to pre-zoned
industrial areas both within and beyond provincial borders. Farmers in
Placid Pond were embedded in these transforming ecologies and economies.
With the money Thủy had saved from working in Taiwan, Thủy and Trí had
been steadily expanding their flock of laying chickens. They started by investing in several hundred commercially bred Egyptian Faiyumi hens. But
although the couple had sufficient funds to change the composition of their
flock and increase its size, they found it difficult to secure enough space to
house the birds. Thủy and Trí did not want to relocate to the larger landholdings that the Vietnamese government had zoned for industrial-integrated
chicken production.[8] As Trí explained, these plots lay on the outskirts of the
village too far removed from familial rice paddies, social networks, and local

markets. Trí added that moving toward industrial farm holdings would also require him to take out loans that would indebt them either to commercial companies or state banks. This was a particularly unappealing prospect for villagers in Placid Pond who were still reeling from the effects of postwar-era state incursions into land use practices. Trí summed it up in this way: "Maybe in America you can go into big business like that and rely on the government, but here in the countryside we like to keep business matters within the home."

Tellingly, Trí used the term *ở trọng nhà* to signify home, a term that collapses concepts of home and family (*nhà* is used to refer to one's house and spouse). Indeed, family was central to the decisions Thủy and Trí made about their productive activities. Instead of relocating to industrial zones, the couple chose to house their expanding flock in the backyards of various relatives, sometimes combining their chickens with their parents' and siblings' flocks, and frequently moving birds between houses scattered around the village before collecting their eggs to sell on the market. At least twice a week Trí would travel over seventy kilometers to neighboring markets, his Taiwanese motorbike weighed down by eggs collected from these various holdings. Depending on the price on any given day, Trí might head north to the provincial market in Lang Sơn, or south to the market in Bắc Giang's industrializing neighbor Bắc Ninh. Or he might sell to a nearby trader or transporter servicing Hanoi city markets. Meanwhile, Thủy directed sales from home, conducting business with itinerant traders who arrived on bicycles or on foot. These traders purchased eggs from several households in the commune and sold them at markets within the commune's borders as well as further afield. Thủy told me that a neighborhood egg peddler in his sixties would sometimes cycle fifty kilometers to Hanoi.

From the perspective of bird flu strategists promoting integrated-industrial farming, Thủy and Trí's production practices were far from ideal: mixing flocks of various origins, breeds, and ages, and moving poultry products short and long distances on foot, bicycle, and motorbike where they exchange all manner of biological materials with humans and other animals. Yet these place-based biological exchanges were common in Vietnam's Red River Delta, and households engaged in a mix of agricultural activities including livestock rearing, rice production, and nut, soy, and fruit farming. The limited land available in this region, coupled with inconsistent market prices for agricultural goods, meant that farmers like Thủy and Trí avoided investing too much in any one activity, preferring instead to draw on kinship and other interpersonal networks to expand their production and sales on their own, private plots.

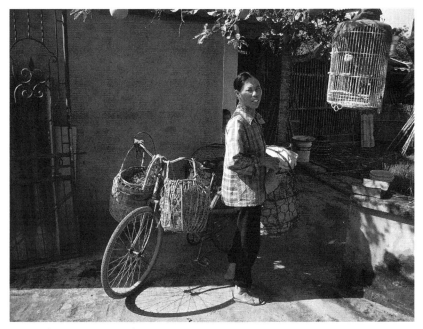

FIG. 5. Itinerant trader on her way to market, where she will sell eggs she has purchased from several household farms. Placid Pond village, Bắc Giang province. Photo by author.

According to livestock analysts, this mixed-method mode of production is popular in many countries in the "developing" world, and represents a transition stage between traditional and commercial poultry (Mcleod, Thieme, and Mack 2009). Such evaluations again point to the naturalizing, evolutionary discourses of modernization and development applied to poultry restructuring in Vietnam and elsewhere. These are powerful discourses. Trí and Thủy themselves believed that their production strategies were more advanced than backyard farming techniques, and Trí often pointed me to the newest antibiotic and commercial feed he was experimenting with.

But while the couple was more or less satisfied with their enterprise, many of their neighbors found their activities offensive. Some of them asked me how I could stand staying at their house. A man who lived over eight hundred meters away remarked, "It's so dirty. Heavens, all those feathers flying. I can smell it from here. They've really polluted the air." During my time in the village, Thủy and Trí's neighbors often invited me over to feast on their backyard chickens, where they would inevitably ask me to compare them to the birds I ate at Thủy and Trí's house (even though Trí and Thủy produced egg-laying hens rather than birds for meat). One neighbor came right out and said:

Their chickens aren't as good, right? Those commercial breeds are tasteless. I guess maybe you Americans like your chicken white and dry but we can't eat that here. Local chicken is smaller and more expensive, but the meat isn't so soft. It's chewy and dark. The meat is stickier. That's how we like it.

Such breed-based distinctions do much to inflect poultry value chains in Vietnam. Throughout my research in Bắc Giang, scores of household producers and their neighbors told me that *gà ta* are not susceptible to bird flu. In the countryside a good, healthy, and tasty chicken is one that has run around in gardens eating plants and insects, not a commercially bred and fed animal common to the cities. Several neighbors warned me against eating the foreign, "Egyptian" chicken cultivated by Trí and Thủy, since some of the larger holdings in the village with commercial breeds had experienced outbreaks of avian pox and fever.

Of course, Thủy and Trí's chickens were not the only life forms under scrutiny. After learning more about the social dynamics and alliances in the village, I realized that those villagers who complained about Thủy and Trí's farm were often those who had fewer resources and social connections within and beyond Placid Pond. On the whole, these villagers had done little to expand their agricultural production arrangements and were not linked up with markets outside of the district. Without the necessary information, techniques, and social contacts for farm expansion (livestock or otherwise), these villagers were less entrepreneurial, less willing to experiment with more productive and profitable forms of life. And they imparted moral judgments on Trí and Thủy by suggesting that their mixed farming methods featured industrial orientations that put rural dwellers at risk. For these neighbors, not quite backyard but not yet industrial farming techniques produced a troubling mix of profit-seeking and parochialism, foreign and domestic life forms. In other words, Trí and Thủy's farm served as a sensory signal that the couple's aspirations were perhaps a bit too high and a bit too outward-looking.

What emerged from Trí and Thủy's experience was a form of poultry production that was increasingly industrious and outward-oriented, but still rooted in a set of kin-based subsistence activities common to northern Vietnam. In the north, poultry is embedded in an agricultural economy where it is complemented by a range of foodstuffs that families have in some sense wrested away from governmental control. Removing fowl from these ecologies was impractical for farmers like Thủy and Trí, who not only relied upon family members to accomplish the daily tasks of mixed agricultural production, but also shied away from commercialization plans that would have them relinquish control of their private plots and rely too heavily on government subsidies or other loans.

Thủy and Trí's poultry production decisions could be explained structurally through James Scott's (1976) notion of the moral economy of the peasant, wherein a "subsistence ethic" precludes risk-taking behavior among inward looking rural dwellers. However, I want to emphasize that the production and marketing practices I observed in Placid Pond signaled aspirations to more than mere subsistence. Thủy and Trí were continually experimenting with ways to change their conditions, maneuvering within an increasingly profitable yet restrictive domestic poultry market to fashion their own kind of future. Thủy's work abroad and the household poultry farm expansion were a few in a series of steps the couple was taking to send their daughter to university in Hanoi. The multispecies exchange relations this family carved out amid viral threats, then, were promissory in nature and dynamic by design, and they relied upon on social arrangements (forms of life) in which people, poultry, and pathogens (life forms) were in constant circulation with other agricultural products, both within and beyond village gates.

Anh

Trí and Thủy were not the only farmers navigating new market dynamics. Some farmers in Placid Pond set their sights even further, and despite contentious histories of state-led agricultural reform, followed the government's encouragement to move to industrial-integrated production zones where they could contract their operations with commercial companies. One farmer, Anh, started a chicken farm in a district about twenty-five kilometers away from Placid Pond. I had become close to Anh's sister, Vy, during my stay in the village. Knowing that I was interested in poultry, one Saturday she invited me to take a trip to Anh's farm. We set out early in the morning to avoid the oppressive tropical heat. Vy's two daughters piled on the back of my motorbike while Vy and her good friend, Sang, climbed onto Sang's newer Honda Wave. Driving was slow but scenic along the bumpy dirt road that led out of the village. Stunning emerald rice paddies, spanning all the way to the imposing Đông Triều mountain range in the distance, flanked our pathway. Vy's daughters were unable to take in the view, however. Unaccustomed to motorized travel they clung to one another and to my sides in an attempt to stay upright. Their grips only tightened as we merged onto the fast-moving highway headed north. As bikes and trucks flew past us, they kicked up a mixture of dust and exhaust into our eyes and nostrils. Vy and Sang, however, took in the reflective storefronts, sleek roadways, and bustling traffic that connected the northern provinces. After about an hour, we turned onto an unpaved path that transected an expanse of razed but not yet developed land. In the distance I glimpsed a concrete building spanning about 100 square meters. This, Vy announced, was Anh's farm.

Anh appeared from behind the compound and greeted us. Tall, built, and tan, he looked younger than his forty-three years. His sparkling, light brown eyes and toothy grin revealed an eagerness to show us around, for this was his sister's first visit and she had brought family and friends. As he guided us to the structure, Anh explained that he was contracting with Thailand's CP agro industrial food conglomerate, which meant that his farm adhered to strict standards for integrated-industrial commercial production. Anh carefully enunciated the technical term "biosafety standards" (*tiêu chuẩn an toàn sinh học*), which made his birds suitable for entry into Hanoi markets.

Poultry farming here took on a very different form than what I had become accustomed to in Placid Pond. Most apparent was the scale of operation. Anh kept about two thousand birds in a state of the art, ventilated coop. In addition to the cement walls, a variety of instruments separated the birds from producers and the elements: a dug-in, paved footbath and a locked entry-gate. Looking inside the coop, I noticed that at four weeks old the homogeneously white birds were already plump and sedentary. Anh's birds congregated in twos and threes around well-spaced, hanging food troughs, and many had lay down on what looked like fresh wood shavings covering the floor.

Anh said that he gave the birds industrial feed (CP brand), which was the only thing that the flock was permitted eat, and that he and his two hired hands vaccinated them regularly for diseases like Marek, Newcastle, and H5N1. I noted that Anh never crossed the threshold of the enclosure, and, unlike other smaller-scale farmers, his descriptions focused not on the fowl and their characteristics, but rather on the infrastructures and devices of the farm—the ventilation system, the concrete edifice, the clean shavings scattered across the floor, and of course, the commercial feed—all components of the integrated and contained, biosecure operation. The chickens remained a visible absence in this farming system. When I said they looked plump he nodded slightly, noting that their weight was on track. Weight. This was a metric I rarely heard uttered from the mouths of farmers, health workers, sure, but not farmers. Plumpness was usually measured by the eye and by touch, by pinching the flanks and pressing against the sides of the bird— not standardized and quantifiable procedures. Absent here was what Susan Squier (2012) calls "fellow feeling," embodied labor practices that produce affect and empathy between farmer and fowl. Care. Anh didn't seem to miss this form of interspecies engagement, however. He beamed at me from the doorway of the enclosure. I looked back inside. The chickens appeared well

ordered, contained, and free of contamination. The extra land and commercial contract seemed to be paying off.

A closer look at Anh's farm, however, signals some of the difficulties involved in adhering to market restrictions, and in relocating poultry away
from family networks and private plots. Though Anh was proud of his farm,
as he walked me around the facilities he confided that the expense of establishing it had put him into debt with relatives. His wife provided much of the
funds for the endeavor (like Thủy had done before, she was working as an au
pair overseas), but he also had to borrow money from close relatives like Vy,
who had just returned from Malaysia where she spent a few years working in
a factory. In addition to these monetary debts, Anh incurred personal ones
as well. Relocating to an industrial farming zone had cost him the ability to
make independent decisions related to land use and poultry production, and
Anh said that it had been difficult to implement CP's commercial standards
with his limited funds and two hired hands.

Industrializing production was not only a struggle for Anh. As we prepared a goose for lunch (a sideline farming occupation to supplement his
commercial production), Vy confided to me that since Anh had left the village she was struggling to keep up with the work on their family's rice paddy.
Her parents were too old to tend to the fields and her husband was still employed in Malaysia, so Vy and her older sister had shared responsibility for
rice cultivation. But when Anh needed extra help on his farm and could not
afford to hire another laborer, Vy's older sister relocated to his plot. Vy was
therefore left to cultivate the family's rice paddy and peanut fields on her
own. Her young daughters had neither the experience nor the strength to
engage in farm labor, and so Vy had to rely on occasional assistance from
friends and in-laws to plant and harvest the fields.

Following official recommendations to integrate and industrialize commercial poultry holdings thus came at a high cost to Anh and his family.
Though he had plugged himself into urban markets, Anh worried that he had
plunged too far into debt to do so. He also lamented his loss of freedom as
an independent farmer, and fretted over the extra labor required to maintain
farm operations on a par with industrial-integrated commercial standards.
Industrialization required hiring day laborers, in whom Anh had little trust,
and whose work he tried to augment with that of his sister. What is more,
Anh's dislocation from his village not only prevented him from assisting with
the rice harvest, but also drew other family members away from this key subsistence activity. And so, although market-oriented disease-control measures
brought Anh new financial opportunities, they also transformed the coopera-

tive kinship networks and land use practices central to agricultural production systems in the north—systems that hinged on poultry's proximity to,
rather than separation from, village households and agrarian space.

Ông Long

Village proximity is rather less critical to poultry production systems in the
southern Mekong Delta, where expansive paddy lands invite free-range
duck-rice farming. As noted, integrated rice-duck production is a common
component of mixed farming systems in the south. Here, ducks are kept in
flocks that scavenge in post-harvest rice fields, and may be moved long distances to follow harvesting patterns. Since the onset of HPAI in Vietnam,
however, health strategists and government officials have argued that these
mobile duck flocks not only ran a high risk of becoming infected from wild
birds and domestic poultry, but they were also poised to spread the disease
to other areas, particularly because ducks are able to remain asymptomatic
for long periods of time (Gilbert et al. 2008). The United States Department
of Agriculture, for instance, estimated that 70 percent of waterfowl in the
Mekong Delta possessed the H5N1 virus. And in 2006 the NSCAI stated that
"populations of grazing ducks [small scale and backyard] should be subject
to compulsory vaccination, movement restrictions and minimization of contact with other poultry . . . [and] where appropriate, upgrading to industrial
production will be encouraged" (National Steering Committee on Human
and Avian Influenza 2006b, 21).

   Restrictions on free-range duck production cycles proved difficult, however. During one of my visits to duck farms in Đồng Tháp province, I met
Ông Long, who owned about two thousand birds—a large flock, but not uncommon in this region. Ông Long had been raising ducks as an independent
farmer for over fifteen years, and he relied upon his extensive contacts to
move his birds in and around the province for feeding before selling them to
a variety of retailers in the region. I asked Ông Long to tell me about how he
raised the animals. He shrugged and said that he followed the typical production pattern, using the local term *bình thường* to emphasize its unexceptional
character. At the start of every planting season, he bought a new flock of
ducklings and then called around to his contacts to inquire about the availability of their rice fields for grazing. After locating a farmer who had not yet
arranged for a flock to occupy his paddy, they would settle on a rental fee for
his ducks to feed at the plot. A few weeks after planting, Ông Long's employees would load the ducks on a boat for transport to the field. Sometimes Ông

Long arranged for the ducks to feed on a plot within Đồng Tháp's borders, while other times he searched as far afield as neighboring provinces or even into Cambodia for a free paddy.

Once they reached the rented paddy, the duck flock would stay at the newly planted field until rice started flowering (approximately twelve weeks), grazing on snails and parasitic insects that attack rice early in the planting season. While feeding, the ducks defecated as they kicked up soil in the process of treading water, serving a bio-commercial function as pest control and nutrient-bearing mechanisms for rice cultivation. After the rice flowered a few weeks later, Ông Long's hired hands would coax the flock through the extensive networks of canals, swamps, and ditches that have defined the Mekong Delta since colonial-era engineering projects transformed the southern ecology (Biggs 2003). All along the way the fattening ducks would feed in the waterways. When the rice grasses grew taller and the ducks got larger, the flocks returned to the paddy fields where they cleared weeds, snails, and crustaceans. After eight to twelve more weeks of fattening, Ông Long would sell the flock to traders who transport the animals by boat to neighboring markets, sometimes as far as Ho Chi Minh City (about sixty-five kilometers to the northeast). He told me that circulating his flocks between paddies had saved him millions of Vietnamese Đồng (several hundred dollars) on commercial feed.[9]

Reflecting what is often characterized as the entrepreneurial spirit of southerners (Salemink 2003), Ông Long's poultry production practices saw him wheeling and dealing with rice producers, traders, and transporters from as far afield as Cambodia. Recalling our conversation, I was reminded of accounts of southern Vietnam that describe how precolonial seafaring and overland trade engendered strong interpersonal networks between and beyond village gates. Ông Long and his ducks inherited a long history of exchange between spatially, ethnically, culturally, and biologically diverse life forms in the region (Taylor 2000). Rather than utilize kin networks to bolster his trade, Ông Long entangled himself and his ducks in a uniquely southern economy that enrolled ducks in spatially expansive landholdings, itinerant labor networks, and entrepreneurial social connections. Duck production in the south required a range of movement far exceeding that of chickens, and it rested on the mobility of hired hands who, just like their precolonial and colonial predecessors, utilized labor rather than land as their primary form of property (Tai and Sidel 2012). Gesturing at his employees, Ông Long joked to me, "These guys are young and single. They can go off for weeks with the ducks. They can even go back to America with you if you like!" Like that of its northern neighbor, southern poultry production was inextricable from rice production. But down south this inextricability had primarily ecological rather than familial overtones. Poultry markets here relied on symbiotic exchanges, and exceedingly *mobile* rice-poultry-human-parasite relations.

The integrative use of space and species in the Mekong Delta was far removed from the contained and circumscribed poultry value chains envisioned by policy makers. One Health strategists soon recognized the importance of the integrated rice-duck production system across Southeast Asia and made policy adjustments to accommodate these mutual ecologies. By 2008, one of the government's primary transnational HPAI collaborators, the FAO, suggested amending containment policies in Vietnam and elsewhere:

> The fact that the flocks move represents a high risk that they could become infected from both wild birds and domestic poultry and spread the disease to other areas. Applying effective biosecurity measures in this system is problematic. The "obvious" answer is to ban free-ranging duck keeping, or to make it socially difficult to continue. But they form an integral part of the "rice/duck" system and the consequences of banning them might be worse than the possible gains. In Thailand, initial restrictions on movement were followed by the provision of resources to house and feed duck flocks. That has been successful, although it may have led to some producers giving up keeping ducks in this system. In Viet Nam, vaccination and some movement control have been used, but the results have not been as good. . . . The identification of practical solutions depends on country-by-country or case-by-case evaluation (Honhold et al. 2008, 51–52).

I quote this report at length in order to show how paramount place is in "global" health, and how open-ended and *multiple* One Health interventions like market restrictions end up becoming. The attention paid in the policy recommendation to the contours of poultry production and virus control in Vietnam's southern ecologies suggests that the country has become an important site for creating and recreating—experimenting with—global strategies against pandemics. The diverse multispecies exchange relations that emerged in the course of this experiment ended up directing future trajectories of disease control, both in Vietnam but also more broadly.

Conclusion

In Vietnam's largest cities, market restrictions aimed to keep certain poultry varieties and their producers on the outskirts of a growing urban consumer base. A combination of targeted quarantines, limitations on value chains, and public rhetoric aligned industrial-integrated commercial poultry with biological safety, and in turn maligned local flocks and their small- and medium-scale producers. Market restrictions thus went beyond the containment of viruses and even market activities to impinge upon people and poultry's forms of life, including their freedom of movement and participation in urban space and social dynamics. And even though such restrictions threatened to push millions of Vietnamese poultry and farmers out of livestock economies altogether, state and multinational strategists cast these endangered life forms and forms of life as necessary collateral damage: the effect of a seemingly natural process of global market integration and economic development. Here again, One Health governance economized life by valuing and preserving the lives of commercial farmers who drive national economic growth, and it did so by encouraging the commoditization of particular kinds of life forms: agro-industrial commercial poultry varieties. Put another way, Vietnam's market restrictions brought epidemiological and economic agendas together in ways that privileged particular places, poultry, and people over others.

Yet the stories presented here reveal that rural dwellers and their poultry were in fact deeply embedded in urban-bound commodity chains, which reflect how difficult it is to define, much less maintain, strict conceptual or material distinctions between city and country in Vietnam.[10] It turns out that poultry are not easily containable commodities; they carry with them biological, economic, and interpersonal attachments, all of which resist disease-control tactics that would limit their exchanges with other life forms. For Trí, Thủy, and Anh in the north, the growth of chicken holdings altered kin-based production practices and redirected the movement of poultry (and its viruses) across different terrains. For Ông Long in the south, the integrated rice-duck farming system called for a synthesis of biological, ecological, and economic exchanges in Vietnamese agriculture—one that pandemic strategists recognized but nevertheless found difficult to accommodate according to principles of market and species containment.

This is not to say that rural-urban distinctions do not carry important meaning in Vietnam. Nhuẩn's comments, mass media messages, and pandemic policy itself indicate the rhetorical force of such differentiations. Nevertheless, in everyday experimental practice individuals broke down and rebuilt these distinctions according to their particular socio-material circumstances and interpersonal obligations. The individuals described here thus illustrate "social edginess," a term Erik Harms (2011) develops to describe how spatial marginalization leaves residents in and around Ho Chi Minh City with a sense of uncertainty: they are indispensable to Vietnam, yet also left out of Vietnam's future-oriented development schemes. Social edginess is an apt descriptor for the poultry farmers described above. At the same time that farmers like Trí, Thủy, Anh and Ông Long struggled to increase production

for an unpredictable and demanding urban market, they were seeing employment opportunities dwindle in light of new industrial and commercial
endeavors concentrated in urban areas and its outliers. Bird flu outbreaks
have taken place in the context of transnational capital flows, which in Vietnam are concentrated in urban centers (Nguyen-Marshall, Drummond, and
Bélanger 2011). Indeed, one of the reasons policy makers chose to experiment
with market restrictions in Hanoi and Ho Chi Minh City was that if they
could establish markets for industrial-integrated commercial poultry in cities, production could then be scaled out for export. In these emerging urban
economies, the life forms and forms of life to which Trí, Thủy, Anh and Ông
Long had become accustomed were becoming less valuable than their industrial counterparts.

But while places like Hanoi and Ho Chi Minh City emerged as new global
markets, transformations in and around these "economic frontiers" have
turned its outlying areas into places of maneuvering and negotiation, sites
where poultry producers engaged in mixed rural and urban, agricultural and
industrial production. Experimentation. In Harm's terms, Thủy, Trí, Anh,
and Ông Long sustained the city while remaining outside of it, though at least
in part on their own terms. And so rural-urban divisions matter. But it is the
particular moments and settings in which they come to matter, and come
apart, that expose the economies in which pandemic planning occurs: economies in which various claims to health and access to markets surface, intersect, and collide. Viruses, then, do not just move with poultry, they move
with people—people who feel particular rights to the products of their labor
and the markets in which to sell them; people who express moral attachments
to one another in their production and consumption practices; people in
symbiotic relations with poultry and other agricultural goods; people who
transect and transcend the social and material spaces and categories to which
they would be contained.

Sacrifice

Vịnh Tranh Gà Lợn
Sáng chưa sáng hẳn, tối không đành
Gà lợn, om sòm rối bức tranh
Rằng vách có tai, thơ có hoa
Biết lòng ai đỏ, mắt ai xanh
Mắt gà huynh đệ bao lần quáng
Lòng lợn âm dương một tấc thành
Cục tác nữa chi, ngừng ủn ỉn
Nghe rồng ngâm váng khúc tân thanh

The Pig and Rooster Painting
Deep in the dark shadows of early dawn
Roosters and pigs bustle in their silk scrolls.
As walls have ears, so verse dissolves in paint.
Who has a pure heart, and who has clear eyes?
How oft is the brotherly rooster blind,
And does the pig's heart see its dream come true?
The cocks stop crowing, the pigs stop oinking,
And the dragon hums its new song to spring.

Penned by acclaimed poet Vũ Hoàng Chương, these verses refer to popular silk scroll paintings that depict pigs and chickens in idyllic village settings (Le 2005). During the Lunar New Year, rural and urban dwellers decorate their homes with these vibrant images to celebrate Vietnam's farming heritage and convey messages of peace and prosperity in the year to come. Throughout the poem, Vũ Hoàng Chương alludes to a number of Vietnamese proverbs and adages pertaining to pigs and roosters, ruminating on their lives and fates as another year springs into being. In doing so, the poet reminds his reader of the prominence of domesticated animals in the Vietnamese imagination.

Livestock, particularly poultry, pervades cultural expression in Vietnam. Poultry surfaces in art, folklore, and moral directives, and figures prominently in ritual practice and leisure activities, shaping ideas about identity and family, nature and culture, human and nonhuman. Here I want to take a closer look at the images, practices, and messages surrounding poultry in Vietnam, and I want to show how these expressions provide idealized moral guides for living and comporting oneself in more-than-human communities. Understanding how poultry-centered images and expressions shape human behavior and attitudes is important because, as I will show, such expressions have long been used to govern populations in Vietnam, and they have found new purpose in bird flu experiments.

I chose *The Pig and Rooster Painting* to highlight poultry's importance to Vietnamese cultural expression in part because the poem references Tết, or Lunar New Year. Marking a new year and a turn to spring, Tết is often described to Americans as Christmas, Easter, Thanksgiving, and everybody's birthday all rolled into one. For weeks leading up to and during the holiday, children sport brand new clothes, designer motorbikes surface on streets in greater number, and beauty salons teem with those seeking a fresh look for the new season. Thousands of gift-bearing citizens assemble at airports, train stations, and bus depots to make the return journey to their home villages, or to welcome loved ones back from afar. Goods pour into shops and households. Festive kumquat trees, red money envelopes, gift-baskets, firecrackers, tea, and liquor occupy storefronts at least one month in advance of the holiday. Poultry, too, abounds, both figuratively and literally.

Like the silk paintings of Vũ Hoàng Chương's prose, folk woodcut paintings from Đông Hồ village in northern Vietnam are ubiquitous during Tết. Long-standing symbols of traditional culture and identity, Đông Hồ paintings depict rural livelihoods as joyous and fruitful, and they often feature livestock, especially poultry, as harbingers of success and well-being. The left-hand image in fig. 6 illustrates distinction (*vinh hoa*) through a young boy's idyllic interactions with a hen, while the right-hand image depicts honor and prosperity (*phú qúy*) in his handling of a plump goose.

Fig. 7, *Gà Đàn*, "Chicken Flock," is a good luck wish. The *Gà Đàn* woodprint is often translated into English as "Chicken Family" because it represents the importance of kinshp ties, especially those between mother and child. A spirited depiction of a mother hen encumbered by the needs of her brood, *Gà Đàn* illustrates a key Vietnamese principle for proper living and comportment: *hy sinh*, or sacrifice. In Vietnamese, *hy sinh* is more encompassing

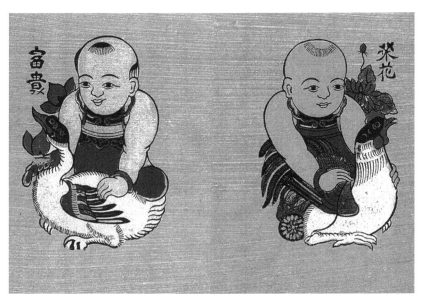

FIG. 6. Đông Hồ folk woodcut paintings. The left-hand image represents distinction, *vinh hoa*, while the right-hand image represents honor and prosperity, *phú qúy*. Source: Available in the Public Domain, from Wikimedia Commons, CC-SA, 3.0, https://commons.wikimedia.org/wiki/File:phú_qúy.jpg.

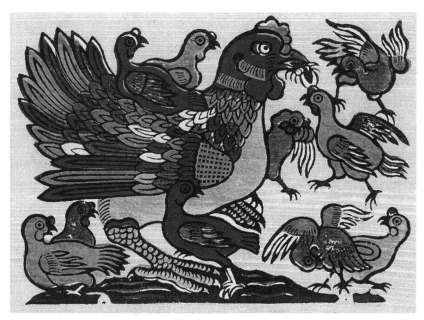

FIG. 7. Đông Hồ folk woodcut painting in which a mother hen tends to her brood. Source: Available in the public domain, from Wikimedia Commons Atlas of the World, CC-SA, 3.0, https://commons.wikimedia.org/wiki/File:Sân_gà.jpg.

than English notions of sacrifice, and has to do with complex obligations and debts that establish and maintain social relations. *Hy sinh* demands that those in lower social positions express filial piety, *hiếu*, by paying respect to their elders through ritual practices and everyday acts of devotion, gratitude, and obedience. It also calls on friends to sacrifice for one another and on citizens to sacrifice for the nation (in times of war and peace). But there is reciprocity here, as *hy sinh* also requires those in higher positions—parents, state authorities, ancestors, teachers, employers—to engage in acts of suffering and accommodation for those with more limited capabilities (Shohet 2013, 212). Importantly, *hy sinh* is an organizing principle for everyday social interactions and exchanges. Ritualized acts of forbearance are sometimes dramatic, but they just as often go unnoticed (Gammeltoft 1998; Nguyen-Vo 2008; Pettus 2003). What's more, *hy sinh* is more than just a practice or behavior. One of its key characteristics is that it is an ethical position animated by strong sentiments and feelings—for family, community, and nation (Shohet 2013, 206). In short, *hy sinh* is an emotive form of life that shapes how individuals understand and experience their place in the social order.

There are many ritualized acts in which poultry support *hy sinh* as a form of life. New Year's celebrations, funerals, death anniversary ceremonies, and weddings almost always feature a boiled, golden-skinned chicken. At these ritual moments, a family will offer a hand-selected, hand-prepared animal to their ancestors, inviting them to join the living for a feast. Most Vietnamese families keep an altar to deceased family members in the house, where they place liquor, fruit, incense, betel nut, and rice in front of photographs of the departed. On special occasions or when asking for spiritual patronage, a chicken is added to family altars. Omitting a chicken in ancestor worship risks offending ancestors, and it must be avoided to uphold virtue. In fact, when the postwar revolutionary government attempted to eliminate spending on ritual accoutrements, villagers responded by continuing to incorporate chicken and other products into ceremonies; their symbolic import and role in maintaining goodwill between living and dead trumped official directives (Malarney 1996).

Because chicken is as popular in the spirit realm as it is in the material realm, the birds are mainstays in rituals that beseech the spirits for blessings. A well-known folk poem relates the story of an unmarried woman who offers a chicken to the deities, Ông Tơ and Bà Nguyệt, an old married couple.

> Em vái Ông Tơ vài ve rượu
> Em cầu bà Nguyệt năm bảy con gà
> Xin cho đôi lứa hiệp hòa
> Rồi sau em xin trả lễ đặng mà đền ơn

I offer Ông Tơ a few bottles of liquor
I pray to Bà Nguyệt with five to seven chickens
Help me find a nice mate
Afterward I'll thank you ceremoniously

Importantly, in these ritual practices, *hy sinh* surfaces in symbolic displays of respect and devotion to the spirits, as well as in the actual physical sacrifice, or slaughter, of the chicken. Killing and preparing a chicken is an evocative, formalized social activity in Vietnam that cements social relations and hierarchies, and creates moral sentiment (*tình cảm*) among people, both living and dead. The procedure begins by slitting the animal's throat and letting the blood slowly drip out, then pouring boiling water over the body while brushing feathers away with bare hands, carefully combing the skin for particularly tenacious plumes. Gutting and partitioning the animal is a meaningful process that reflects biosocial relations between people and poultry. The bird is divided among family members according to their structural position in the family, with the neck and head going to the household patriarch, the body and wings to women and younger men, the feet to children, and the vital organs to those who might be ill and in need of some extra blood or protein. Women often work together when slaughtering, chatting as they prepare the fowl for feasting. Though it is a time for socialization, the skill and attention that a woman brings to the slaughtering process is critical, since her relatives may be watching closely to evaluate whether she will prepare a bird suitable for consumption. A woman's bodily postures and comportment around poultry, much like the children in the Đông Hồ images, reflect her moral subjectivity, or virtuousness.

The 2000 film, *The Vertical Ray of the Sun* (*Mùa Hè Chiều Thẳng Đứng*), illustrates the gendered practices that bring chickens and humans together in meaningful sacrifices that sustain the family and please ancestral spirits. I use a film to discuss this physical-spiritual exchange because it illustrates the evocative force of chicken imagery in Vietnam, something that has become important to bird flu messaging. This film includes a scene depicting a death anniversary ceremony, in which three sisters pay remembrance to their beloved mother. It begins with an up-close image of the golden contours of a chicken thigh, though the magnification is so intense it is unclear what the viewer is looking at. All she sees is a golden, dewy, undulating yellow landscape lightly scored by a repeating triangle pattern. The camera then passes over the body, revealing a ray of sun peeking through the small gap between the chicken's neck and its body. The frame zooms out onto an image of a fully intact, newly slaughtered chicken. The bird is large; the body almost spills over the edges of the gleaming white platter on which it is perched. The hind-quarters are angled upward and its wings point forward and out. The bird's face points skyward, out into the distance as if ready to take flight.

The three sisters inspect the chicken carefully. Their own faces, also gleaming and dewy, are just inches from the animal's body. Drops of sweat around their hairlines mirror the drops of condensation collecting on the chicken's saffron-colored skin. Bodies are entangled; human and nonhuman skins mutually react to a shared environment, sweating and gleaming in harmony. As the sisters look for blemishes, their faces come so close to the bird's body it seems as though their noses will brush against the beads forming on its skin. It is important for the women to get up close, though, for the condition of the bird will say a lot to their mother about how capable they are, how much they value her, and whether or not they deserve her blessing. The sisters' eyes eventually meet over the body and the eldest declares, "Wonderful, there's no damage anywhere on the skin."

The scene then switches to the image of a solid teak altar featuring a large photograph of the mother. In front of the altar stands a table filled with dishes of food. On the altar itself are the higher-value items, incense, betel nut, and the chicken, in whose mouth the women have placed a single pink flower. Then comes a montage with each family member, from eldest to youngest, praying at the altar. At the conclusion of each prayer, before bowing and moving away, the living descendant gazes straight ahead, and the chicken, incense, and ancestral image stand clearly in their line of sight. When it is time to eat, the sisters serve their husbands and male relatives first and then dine later at a separate table.

In this short film segment, the viewer witnesses how the preparation of poultry offerings, the sequence of ritualized prayer, and the spatio-temporal patterns of chicken consumption reinforce kin and gender hierarchies. Throughout all of these activities, women engage in visible and invisible sacrifices or forbearances that mediate relations between the living and dead: they toil and sweat, they inspect, they prepare and then forgo food, and they pray. Chicken is indispensible to these sacrificial acts of piety and patronage, as their surrendered lives unite the cosmos and maintain the social order.

Taken together, these cultural expressions—ritualized spirit offerings, folk poems, and art—convey meaningful exchanges between people and poultry that both reflect and solidify social relations on earth (âm) as well as in heaven (dương). Some of these exchanges are invisible and inexpressible, while others are not; some rely on intercorporeal interactions, while others are more figurative in form. In all of these expressions, poultry connect bodies and worlds through ideals of filial piety and sacrifice. In turn, these connections and exchanges shape health, virtue, and well-being. With such cultural and ideological force behind them, it is not surprising that poultry-centered imagery and messages have provided excellent tools for governing populations, for the purposes of nationalist development, economic modernization, and, most recently, bird flu control. I turn now to these poultry-centered tools of governance.

4

Marketing Morals

Ba mẹ yên tam
Con còn nhỏ lắm
Gia cầm lây bệnh
Con không chạm vào

For parents' peace of mind
You must remember
When poultry get sick
Don't touch

Kìa bé giỏi ngoan
Một điều cần nhớ
Chẳng may bị lỡ
Chạm vào gia cầm
Rửa tay xà phòng
Để hết mầm bệnh

Obedient children
Remember this trick
Don't forget
When you have touched poultry
Wash your hands with soap
To get rid of germs

Gia cầm nhà nuôi
Giúp tăng thu nhập
Nhưng cần phải được bảo đảm an toàn
Con khỏe, con ngoan
Gia đình hạnh phúc

Này các bạn ơi
Nói cùng bạn khác điều mình vừa học
Giúp cho mọi người

Household poultry keeping
Helps increase income
But always watch out for safety
Healthy, obedient children
Make happy families
Hey friends
Share what you've learned
Help for everyone

Under the auspices of responsible parenting, filial piety, and community safety, the rhyming messages in UNICEF's illustrated *Pocket Poultry Guide* exhort farmers and their children to discipline themselves in their various exchanges with poultry. In the ideal-type behaviors promoted here, obedient, responsible children mind their parents by controlling their contact with livestock, and conscientious farmers teach their families and their neighbors how to stave off infection. These behaviors not only promise disease prevention, but they also guarantee increased income, family happiness, and moral standing.[1]

Almost immediately after the H5N1 virus first surfaced in Vietnamese

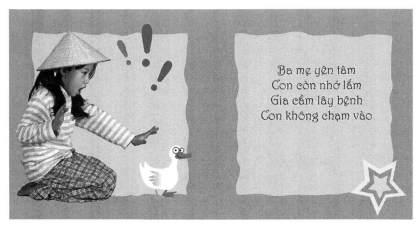

FIG. 8. "For parents' peace of mind you must always remember not to touch sick or dead poultry." This image appeared in a leaflet entitled, "Pocket Poultry Raising Guide" (*Bài Học Hôm Nay: Về Chăn Nuôi Gia Cầm*). Source: Avian Influenza Communications Resources, UNICEF. Reprinted with permission from UNICEF.

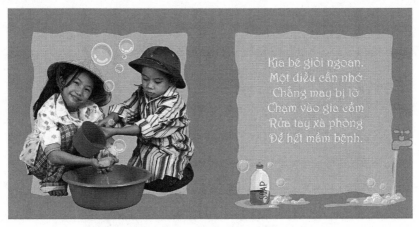

FIG. 9. "Obedient children remember this trick. When you've had contact with poultry wash your hands with soap to get rid of germs." This image appeared in a leaflet entitled, "Pocket Poultry Raising Guide" (*Bài Học Hôm Nay: Về Chăn Nuôi Gia Cầm*). Source: Avian Influenza Communications Resources, UNICEF. Reprinted with permission from Unicef.

poultry, informational messages began to appear on billboards, in newspapers, on television programs, over village loudspeakers, and on radio spots and public service announcements. Initially, these messages aimed to raise awareness of H5N1's existence and convey information about the virus's infection routes. As bird flu became endemic to domestic poultry, the messages changed their focus from raising awareness to shaping behaviors. That is, they began encouraging citizens to adopt new practices to prevent disease transmission, and to abandon existing practices that facilitate it.

Such persuasive messaging falls under the banner of behavior change communications (BCC), a health intervention often associated with neoliberal principles of governance. Drawing on Michel Foucault, theorists suggest that neoliberal governing centers on the conduct of conduct: regulating and modifying behaviors so that individuals can act more effectively in market economies (Foucault 1991, 87–104; Li 2007; Rose 2006). Neoliberal governance follows market logics; it favors cost-efficient, technical management techniques, and is preoccupied with assessing their results (Strathern 2000). In public health, such logics give rise to interventions that promote cheap and measurable modifications to bodily practices. Rather than address the ecological or structural factors that affect health, behavior change communications links health outcomes to concrete actions like hand washing, which can be achieved at very little cost—even less than quick fixes like vaccination. There is a moral dimension to this form of governing, and BCC promotes behaviors as models for correct, modern, and civilized personhood. Put simply, behavior change appeals to people as rational health consumers who "buy into," or choose, healthy behaviors as part of an ongoing project of self-regulation and self-improvement.

For many theorists, interventions like behavior change mark a paradigm shift in health care: whereas state governments were once responsible for providing health services, under neoliberalism individuals care for themselves as responsible health consumers (Defossez 2016). In Vietnam, where there is a long tradition of state-controlled, socialized health care, scaling back the role of government can appear particularly paradigm shifting (Fritzen 2007; Chen and Hiebert 1994). HPAI programmers in Hanoi perceived such shifts, and when the NSCAI promoted behavior change communications for bird flu, they worried that citizens would continue to lean on state-subsidized services like mass vaccination and hygiene inputs. Programmers also worried that citizens would be incapable of choosing healthy behaviors for themselves because they were used to officials telling them what to do. For these programmers, behavior change communications would be a far-reaching, experimental intervention. In addition to reordering people-poultry relations, behavior change would transform how Vietnamese populations could be governed in the future.

For their part, anthropologists have been wary of totalizing narratives which suggest that neoliberalism radically departs from other forms of managing populations and population health. They point out that in countries with socialist legacies, statist national institutions and forms of governance do much to shape neoliberal agendas (Kipnis 2008; Gainsborough 2010). In an analysis of research from Vietnam, Christina Schwenkel and Ann Marie Leshkowich (2012) note that neoliberalism is neither hegemonic nor monolithic; rather, it consists of diverse practices and institutions that are informed by local cultures and histories. Following Aihwa Ong (2006), Schwenkel and Leshkowich propose that we pay attention to exceptional sites where neoliberal forms of governing are seen as new, unusual, or problematic. Experimental. The challenge for the anthropologist, then, is to trace how *multiple* governing logics and practices intersect as Vietnam transitions to market-oriented socialism (Schwenkel and Leshkowich 2012, 380).

I now take up this challenge by exploring an exceptional, experimental moment in which behavior change communications were introduced to Vietnamese public health programs for HPAI. Instead of assuming that BCC constituted a neoliberal rupture to existing governing techniques, I compare behavior change messaging with socialist era propaganda to identify continuities between different styles of managing populations in Vietnam. I argue that both socialist mass mobilization and HPAI communications used artistic depictions of virtuous sacrifice (*hy sinh*) and the technoscientific management of livestock to regulate behavior. I further suggest that these continuities have important implications for how we understand neoliberalism and global health more broadly. First, the ideal of self-responsibility, so commonly associated with neoliberalism's emphasis on the individual, surfaced within a Vietnamese cultural idiom of sacrifice for family, community, and nation. In Vietnam, the responsibilized health subject is embedded in social relations with other humans and animals—she is a person who acts responsibly *for others*. Second, the rational, technoscientific management of health problems is not unique to neoliberal governance, but rather overlaps with socialist uses of science as a means to modernize livestock production and improve lives. Behavior change communications actually extend a historical process in which industrialized life forms and forms of life have been deemed more valuable than others. Experiments to economize life that began in the socialist era have found new expression in a pandemic era. In other words, BCC engages with existing ways of conducting conduct in Vietnam, and exposes the enduring influence of nation-states and cultural values in global health.

I begin by reading bird flu media messages against revolutionary-era propaganda posters. Here I highlight how BCC resonates with a national discourse that (1) encourages sacrifice for family and nation as a virtuous practice, and (2) celebrates scientized multispecies exchanges as avenues toward human development and enlightened nation building. I then ethnographically trace how one behavior change campaign developed communications messages. I detail how state and multinational health workers experimented with ways to combine social marketing, participatory development, and mass mobilization techniques in order to establish healthy behaviors as consumer products. Symbols of family responsibility, community accountability, and rationalized livestock production, which the government has long used to manage populations, found particular purchase in this experiment. Self-regulation emerged in this health intervention as yet another form of sacrifice—for family, farms, and fatherland.

Since the onset of avian flu outbreaks, the government of Vietnam (with support from the UN, multilateral agencies, bilateral donors, and NGOs) has been using health communications to raise public awareness of HPAI circulation, and to impart recommendations for disease control. In 2006, the National Steering Committee on Human and Avian Influenza (NSCAI) stated:

Control strategies must include awareness raising and public information and behavior change campaigns. It is extremely important to raise and maintain awareness in the public and private sectors, to address behavior changes in the medium/long term and to strengthen coordination mechanisms for the implementation of the necessary technical responses, involving the Government, the donor community, the private sector, and civil society (National Steering Committee on Human and Avian Influenza 2006b, 4).

In this statement, the NSCAI posits awareness raising as a first-phase response against HPAI, which will pave the way for longer-term behavior change campaigns. Awareness raising employed a one-way process of communication that sought first and foremost to relay information to mass audiences via state-run television, newspapers, radio broadcasts, billboards, and leaflets. Informational messages focused on describing interspecies transmission routes and disease symptoms, and identifying risky spaces and bodies.

As awareness-raising messages circulated throughout the country, the NSCAI was developing a longer-term and more robust communications strategy to respond to the evolving HPAI situation in Vietnam. In 2008, the NSCAI published the *National Strategic Framework for Avian and Human Influenza Communications*, known among HPAI strategists as "The Gray Book." The Gray Book calls for multinational communications activities to provide the public with clear, consistent, technically sound, and feasible messages that align with specific goals for behavior change (National Steering Committee for Human and Avian Influenza 2008, 3). The Gray Book evaluated 184 proposed behavioral outcomes to prevent H5N1 exposure and ranked them according to technical relevance (efficacy in preventing virus infection and transmission) and practical feasibility (the likelihood that target groups would adopt the behavior). From these rankings, the Gray Book delineated twenty "priority behavioral outcomes" targeting communities where humans lived in close proximity with poultry. In 2008, the Gray Book was disseminated to all of the UN agencies, NGOs, research centers, non-profit, and for-profit firms with HPAI programs in the country, as well as to all provincial, district, commune, and village-level Communist Party headquarters and human and animal health agencies. By the time I began research in Hanoi, most foreign donors and multinational organizations in bird flu management had begun to develop campaigns in accordance with the Gray Book's priorities for behavior change. I will provide an ethnographic examination of one of these campaigns in the pages that follow. First, I want to give some historical context for these types of communications campaigns.

Life Imitates Art: The Aesthetics of Governing in Vietnam

Health communications for disease control hinge on social mobilization, which has a unique history in Vietnam. Scholars of international health development describe social mobilization as a process that raises awareness of particular social objectives (such as disease prevention) and motivates populations toward achieving those objectives. The website of one of its key proponents, UNICEF, states that social mobilization seeks to empower communities to fight disease by providing avenues for them to take ownership over their health and health behaviors. But social mobilization has other connotations, too. Also known as mass or popular mobilization, social mobilization refers to processes that motivate populations toward political (often revolutionary) ends. This type of mobilization can also be couched as an empowering endeavor, and frequently surfaces in independence movements. These two forms of social mobilization intersected in Vietnamese HPAI communications, particularly in media messages and imagery.

Vietnamese leaders have long used art as tool to encourage citizens to conduct themselves in accordance with national directives, particularly in times of uncertainty and political transformation. After Hồ Chí Minh declared independence from French colonizers in 1945, and until the end of the Second Indochina War in 1975, Vietnam was split into two states: the Democratic Republic of Vietnam (DRV) in the North, and the Republic of Vietnam (RVN) in the South. In 1950, in the midst of the First Indochina War against the French, leaders of the DRV founded a Propaganda Posters Bureau under the Department of Information and Propaganda.[2] They recruited Vietnamese artists into a cadre of "state art workers" assigned to promote a "national character" that exemplified the spirit of a Vietnamese people struggling for independence. In a 1951 exhibition, DRV President Hồ Chí Minh told artists:

> Literature and art are also a fighting front. You are fighters on this front. Like other fighters, you combatants on the artistic front have definite responsibilities: to serve the Resistance, the Fatherland, the people, first and foremost the workers, peasants, and soldiers . . . get in close touch with and go deeply into the people's life (Ho Chi Minh 2001 [1951], 133).[3]

The DRV advocated socialist realism as the new national art genre and the only state-sanctioned form of expression for newly politicized artists. Socialist Realism is a style of theory and composition in literature and art developed in the Soviet Union and adopted in various other countries to further the goals of socialism and Communism.[4] Socialist Realist paintings and sculptures used naturalistic and idealized imagery to portray workers and farmers as dauntless, purposeful, forward looking, and powerful. Future oriented. Meant for mass consumption, propaganda also drew in audiences by incorporating familiar artistic conventions, including features of Vietnamese folk art (such as the heavy lines and rich colors of Đông Hồ woodblock printing), and traditional imagery associated with happiness and prosperity such as domesticated animals, lush crops, and national heroes. In addition to these artistic conventions, socialist propaganda also recapitulated existing cultural ideas and moral precepts to further appeal to viewers (Heather and Buchanan 2009, 10–13).

SECURITY THROUGH SACRIFICE

Thematically, propaganda art promoted a national narrative in which the family comprised the metonymical representation of the nation, as well as the primary unit of social organization and mobilization. It gained traction by drawing on timeworn understandings of the role of parents (especially mothers) as sacrificial household guardians. As Vietnamese art ethnographer Nora Taylor notes,

> [Propaganda] alluded to the nation as a "house" where people lived under the same "roof." The nation as a home was also illustrated in posters with images of women, or mothers. The family being an important aspect of Vietnamese society, in drawing a parallel between the nation as head of the people and the mother as head of a household, these posters provided a definition of nationalism that every citizen could understand (2004, 60).

In a time of political uncertainty and transformation, state-sanctioned art depicted the family household as a symbol of the nation in need of protection. Propaganda was thus a gendered social mobilization effort, one that drew on a historical cultural tradition which cast women as "generals of the home" (*nội tướng*) responsible for maintaining family well-being (Turner 1999). Historian Hue-Tam Ho Tai observes, "The representation of war as an exercise in patriotic self-defense makes possible its feminization. It makes use of images of a country as victim of oppression and as family whose home is being invaded" (Tai 2001, 173).[5]

Women's social mobilization was couched in the rhetoric of sacrifice, or *hy sinh*, for family and nation. In addition to protecting their children, mothers were encouraged to give them up to the revolutionary cause. As Hồ Chí Minh declared, "Our people is grateful to the mothers, of both North and South, who have given birth to and raised all the generations of heroes for our country" (Tai 2001, 170). Sacrifice is an important virtue in Vietnam that draws from both Confucian and Buddhist precepts, and women especially are expected to forgo many things for the well-being of their family (see Pettus 2003). In return, children are expected to respect their parents by acting obediently. According to Merav Shohat, this "disposition to sacrifice" is socialized among family members from a very early age: routine directives and bodily actions repeatedly emphasize adults' accommodation to children, and children's compliance to elders (Shohet 2013, 212). As historian David Marr summarizes, "Vietnamese tradition abounded with mothers who made endless sacrifice for their sons, especially the eldest, and with men who were motivated . . . by the desire to repay maternal kindness" (Marr 1981, 198).

Artistic expression in Vietnam conveys the theme of sacrificial mother. Fig. 10 shows a smiling mother with an infant in one hand and a gun in the other. The message reads, "For our future." The look on the mother's face is determined and optimistic, as if she is contemplating a bright tomorrow for herself and her child. The stylized rice grains in the background are telling, since messages at the time encouraged women to forsake their family farms and take up arms for the revolution. Family sacrifice is contiguous with national sacrifice because it is done in the name of a collective future that is personified by the sleeping child. The viewer can expect that the young child will someday be a sacrificial person—that this scene will be repeated in generations to come. As Patricia Pelley argues, revolutionary rhetoric naturalized national struggle as continuing the past into the present, especially in the image of women as primordial defenders of a home repackaged as the nation (Pelley 2002, 181).[6]

RATIONALIZING RISKS

Ideals of virtuous sacrifice found expression in the Cultured Family Campaign (*Gia Đình Văn Hoá*), which has been a key technique of mass mobilization since the Second Indochina War. Originally associated with agricultural collectivization in the DRV in 1962, the Cultured Family Campaign promoted collective labor, good hygiene, and conformity to Communist Party policies. In the early decades of Communist governing, images of cultured families played a decisive role in promoting socialist modernity (Drummond and Rydstrøm 2004, 164–65). Key themes centered on modernizing agriculture to sustain families, support the war effort, and rebuild a nation devastated by battle. Propaganda posters from the socialist era can still be found today in souvenir shops all over Vietnam. One popular image, fig. 11, brings symbols of family together with those of productive farming. In the foreground, a

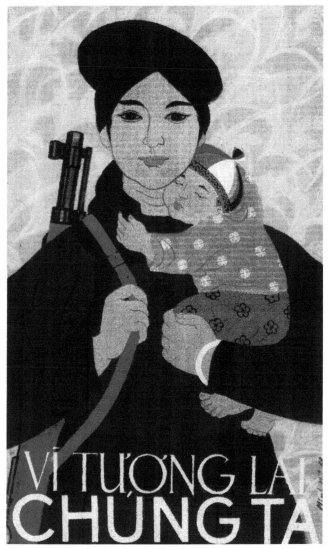

FIG. 10. "For our future." Propaganda poster encouraging women to take up arms. Reprinted poster owned and reproduced by author.

young girl feeds a family of chickens that have been lined and colored in a way that resembles the chicken flock in the Đông Hồ woodcut, *Gà Đan* (see fig. 7). In the background, the girl's fellow villagers engage in various other industrious activities. The image conveys the collective being promoted by the state at the time. As the people in the background head off to their rice paddies, vegetable gardens, and schoolhouses, the viewer gets a strong sense of community and cooperation. Governance here is future-oriented. It combines economics and aesthetics in the message "For a rich and beautiful Vietnam."

Importantly, Vietnam's future prosperity was tied to industrialization. Long before market-oriented *đổi mới* reforms, the DRV was engaged in a Marxist-Leninist inspired project to standardize and industrialize agricultural production. In a 1960 speech delivered at a meeting for the commemoration of Lenin's ninetieth birthday, Lê Duẩn, general secretary of the Communist Party, defined Vietnam's industrialization policy as one that aimed to

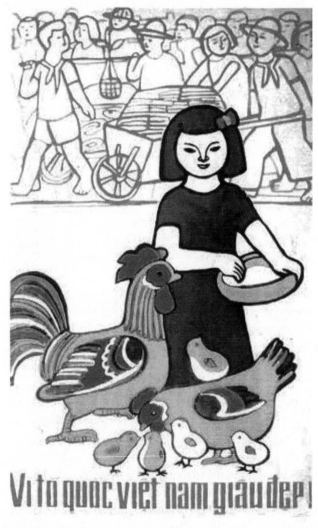

FIG. 11. "For a rich and beautiful Vietnam." Propaganda poster encouraging agricultural labor and chicken production. Reprinted poster owned and reproduced by author.

build a balanced and modern socialist economic structure in coordinating industry with agriculture, to take industry as a foundation, in giving priority to its rational development, at the same time to strive to develop agriculture and light industry with a view to turning our backward country into a socialist one endowed with modern industry and modern agriculture (Porter 1979, Document 27, 68–70).

Idealized images of science and agriculture pervaded propaganda posters, where they obtained local cultural expression. Livestock, long-standing symbols of family health, happiness, and prosperity, were incorporated into pictures of rational, scientific production. Recall fig. 1, which exhorts viewers to "Develop Chicken Production." Large, homogenous-looking chickens surround a woman, who carries a bucket and wears an apron to mark her professionalism. Similar messages included images of ordered, industrial chicken coops, replete with hanging feed and water sources, contained spaces, and identical, alert birds. Pigs, too, appeared in propaganda. Fig. 12 uses an image of a mother, son, and gargantuan pig to encourage viewers to diversify rice farming with industrial animal husbandry and crop production. Other propaganda images exhorted scientific production practices by depicting lab-coated professionals alongside villagers and salutary sows (Heather and Buchanan 2009, 177). Such images indicate that science and industry result in increased productivity as well as family and community well-being.

Health prescriptions also surfaced in messages that linked disease control to state strength and social development. Posters frequently promoted vaccination, or "hygienic inoculation" of livestock to protect against epidemics (Heather and Buchanan 2009, 213). When put in historical context, inoculation says a lot about the use of science, industry, and public health for socialist state development. In his study of malaria control measures, Michitake Aso (2013) develops the concept of "patriotic hygiene" to show how knowledge about malaria was produced within the context of larger health and political concerns of the DRV. Aso details how DRV propaganda made use of scientific imagery and language to encourage citizens to rationalize human-nonhuman interactions. Strategies of patriotic hygiene were meant to combat backwardness as well as disease, and comprised attempts to introduce civilized ideas to rural northern Vietnam as part of a broader strategy of nation building.[7]

Similarly, Shaun Malarney has shown how public health campaigns at the time spread knowledge about germ theory, and encouraged villagers to eliminate "unscientific" (*phản khoa học*) and "unhygienic" (*phan vệ sinh*) agricultural practices to combat malaria. A first step was to rebuff disease understandings that tied malaria to miasma, pollution, toxicity, and ghosts,

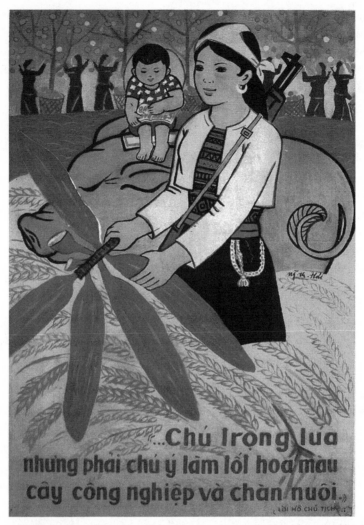

FIG. 12. "Focus on rice production, but pay attention to making good industrial crops and livestock." Propaganda poster encouraging the industrialization of livestock and other agricultural goods. Reprinted poster owned and reproduced by author.

and convince villagers that poisonous mosquitoes carried the germ. A second step was to introduce hygiene measures that mediated human-nonhuman animal relations through technical intervention (2012, 111). Much like international health development workers today, patriotic health planners worked under the assumption that transforming villagers' knowledge and attitudes about disease transmission would lead to transformations in hygiene and health improvements.

The images and messages of patriotic hygiene and agricultural modernization signal that the use of science to address health and development problems has a long genealogy in Vietnam. As early as the revolutionary period, Vietnamese leaders have treated social issues as technical problems best solved by the state and its cadre of scientific experts, and they have engaged in an ideological campaign that values industrialization and modernization over other forms of life. State efforts to economize life gained cultural credibility in propaganda that linked industrialization and modernization to family health and prosperity, and that deployed idealized images of livestock, which have long been associated with the good life and moral comportment in Vietnam.

FLOCKS, FAMILY, AND FATHERLAND

Images of sacrificial, cultured, and modern families have adjusted to changing political-economic conditions in Vietnam. As the country transitions to a market economy with socialist orientation, the Cultured Family has shifted from a model of nationalist, socialist citizenship to a model of family quality. Improved emotional relations, material conditions, and civic engagement have become the new benchmarks of cultured families (Leshkowich 2014, 143). The tenor and content of *hy sinh* has also shifted to meet these benchmarks. During and immediately after the wars, sacrifice meant mobilizing for national liberation and economic modernization. Today, in the context of peace and rising prosperity, sacrifice has come to mean cultivating good family relations and mastering the ways *and perils* of the market economy (Shohet 2013, 212). The threats to families shift, but the need for vigilance remains constant.

How do such ideals translate to HPAI communications? A calendar developed by UNICEF's Avian Influenza Communications division includes an awareness-raising message for each month of the year. The month of July (fig. 13) depicts a family whose conical hats, sandals, and military garb index their rural lifestyle. The father holds up a chicken by its feet. The animal's rich coloring and lush feathers indicate good health. This poster reads, "Their lives are in your hands" (*Cuộc sống của họ nằm trong tay bạn*), referring literally to the chicken whose life is in the hands of the farmer, and figuratively to the girls for whom he is responsible. While the poster uses the term *cuộc sống* to index life, *hy sinh* sacrifice also has connotations related to life. *Sinh* is often found in lexical compounds relating to life, living, and giving birth (Shohet 2013, 205). One can imagine Vietnamese viewers making connections between virtuous acts of family sacrifice and the protection of life against avian flu. Remember, too, that sacrifice goes both ways, and in this

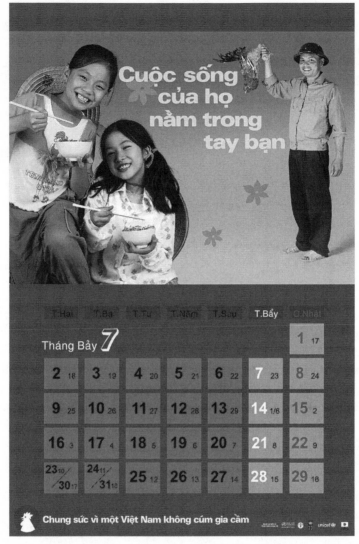

FIG. 13. "Their lives are in your hands." Image from a 2007 bird flu calendar. Source: Avian Influenza Communications Resources, Unicef. Reprinted with permission from UNICEF.

poster children comport themselves properly. The daughters smile into the camera, demonstrating their filial piety and obedience by the proper way in which they clutch their chopsticks and rice bowls.

A series of television spots developed by the Government–UN Joint Program on Avian and Human Pandemic Influenza shows parents embracing healthy behaviors as a means to protect their family and to promote more modern, rational forms of life. One spot employs satirical images of rural peasants to warn against eating sick or dead poultry. It begins with a visage of a quiet village lane accompanied by a peculiarly Asian sounding xylophonic percussion riff. The camera zooms in on a man sporting an expansive grin and the brown cotton pajamas and conical hat common to peasant farmers. In his left hand he holds the reins for his water buffalo, and with his right hand he pats his companion animal as he heads down the path leading to his thatched roof home. As he ties the buffalo to a post and sets down his plowing tools, he looks askance and spots a dead chicken in the garden. "Uả," he asks, surprised, "Whose chicken died in our garden?" Then, with a smile, he declares that the family will feast on delicious meat tonight. Breaking into a jig, he calls for his wife, who enters the garden with a pleasant grin on her face. Her smile turns in to a scowl, however, when she sees the chicken.

"I bet you're craving chicken tonight."

Still smiling, her husband answers, "Our family hasn't had a chicken meal for a long time!"

"But this is a dead chicken, honey." The camera zooms in on her face so that she is addressing the viewer and her husband simultaneously. "To prevent bird flu we mustn't have direct contact with sick or dead poultry. What's more, when we see sick or dead or dead poultry, we should notify local authorities immediately."

"Really?" her husband asks, the camera zooming in on his enlightened face. "Well then, let's notify the authorities."

The camera then captures the couple standing side by side in front of their home with their thumbs in the air. Together they tell the viewer, "Work together for a bird flu-free Vietnam!"

The smart, hard-nosed woman in this TV spot can be seen as a contemporary manifestation of the female household general lauded in socialist mass mobilization propaganda. She shows affection toward her husband and is responsible and protective to a fault. Though her family hasn't eaten chicken for a long time, this woman makes calculated decisions about the disease risks contained in the dead bird's body, and engages in an act of sacrificial forbearance that protects her loved ones from infection. There are some important cultural and moral tropes operating in this segment, for while the images of the village are peaceful and idyllic, they are also patronizing. The corny music and the buffoonish farmer reflect stereotypes about the backwardness and lack of hygiene in rural settings. But the message is ultimately one of hope, promising a future in which knowledge can uplift and civilize even the most ignorant, uncultured family members. The woman in the segment is a rational role model *and consumer*, educating her husband and viewers of each and everyone's responsibility to keep families, and nation, disease free.

A second TV spot projects similar themes onto urban settings. The segment begins again with Asian-themed background music. A man dressed in a tailored suit and tie walks through his sparkling, utterly modern home. The wooden floors and recessed lighting literally glow as he steps into a kitchen and encounters his wife. Her hair is dyed an orange-blond color popular among urban dwellers, and it is perfectly styled in large curls that fall over her collared blouse and apron.

"What are you doing honey?" her husband asks.

"I'm making your favorite chicken salad," she answers, deftly shredding fully cooked chicken with *gloved* hands.

"What a capable housewife!"

"Of course, dear, because health is precious. I even bought the vaccinated chicken. Consuming vaccinated poultry reduces the risk of bird flu." The image switches to a plated chicken whose drumstick is stamped with a blue vaccine certificate.

The camera then pans out to a view of the couple smiling as they look into the camera. They inform the viewer, "For the sake of your health and your family's health, you should only use healthy and vaccinated poultry." They then strike the same thumbs-up pose. "Work together for a bird flu–free Vietnam!"

This TV spot adjusts the theme of virtuous parents to the tastes of urban audiences. In Vietnam's largest cities, HPAI measures require that poultry sold in markets be industrially produced, processed, and vaccinated. The woman in this video lives in an increasingly prosperous, market-oriented society, and while she seems to have achieved the wealth and beauty her predecessors strove for, she must nevertheless remain vigilant. And so, in accordance with the Cultured Family Campaign's contemporary agenda to foster more affective family relations, material prosperity, and civic duty, this loving housewife uses the trappings of modern life (hygienic gloves, vaccinated meat, a well-apportioned home) to protect her family and country from the negative consequences of economic growth and commodification (Leshkowich 2012, 502). In this short clip, an economization of life that values modern, rational forms of living goes hand in hand with the commoditization of certified industrial and vaccinated poultry life forms.

These media messages reveal important continuities about the ways that people have been governed in Vietnam over time. In his study of HIV/AIDS, Alfred Montoya argues that the subject of health interventions has shifted. Socialist techniques that governed "the people" (*nhân dân*) against aggressing enemies have given way to neoliberal techniques that govern humanity against more elusive disease agents. He suggests that HIV/AIDS interven-

tions operate in an economy of virtue, in which individual bodily discipline
protects a globally abstracted human, rather than a concrete social collective (2012, 572). Governance works differently with regard to bird flu. The
subject of HPAI messaging is thoroughly socially embedded—primarily in
families, but also in communities and nations—and individual bodily discipline is virtuous *insofar* as it protects these social collectives. What's more,
these collectives are tangible and familiar, and it is significant that HPAI messages make little or no reference to more abstract ideas about global health
or the global common good. And so although pandemic flu threats have inspired countless stories of global devastation, and inspired a One World One
Health rhetoric of global humanitarian crisis, in Vietnam, bird flu communications are self-consciously local and national. Like socialist propaganda,
BCC takes the family as the unit of social mobilization, and posits the family,
and by symbolic extension the nation, as the primary beneficiaries of health
intervention.

Reading revolutionary era propaganda against contemporary HPAI communications also demonstrates the enduring role of art and visual media in
disciplining subjects. Mass media has long been used to inculcate desires
for particular practices and forms of personhood, and this is especially true
in Communist settings (Rofel 2007). In Vietnam, socialist propaganda and
HPAI messages both employ a regime of words and images that speak to culturally salient social structures and moral sentiments, whether in the form of
sacrificial family members or the scientific management of livestock. By traf-
ficking in such aesthetic conventions, bird flu messages resonate with sedimented notions about how to engender well-being and social advancement
in Vietnam.

In launching this comparison, I do not mean to suggest that HPAI communications has seamlessly adopted socialist state mobilization devices to its
own ends. Doing so would ignore decades of social, political, and economic
transformations in the country that have altered the role of the Vietnamese
state in everyday moral direction. Doing so would also ignore on-the-ground
negotiations over how to govern through communication in a context of
emerging risks. I turn now to such negotiations.

Hearts, Minds, and Handwashing

As multinational organizations take a more prominent role in Vietnamese
health care, didactic modes of social mobilization have come into contact
with an increasingly development- and market-oriented landscape of global
health programming. Over the last thirty years, approaches to health com-

munication in resource poor settings have shifted from a one-way, "doctor's orders" model toward more interactive programs that cater to at-risk communities' tastes, capabilities, and desires. Against this backdrop, social marketing and participatory development have become the most influential strategies in the field of health communication. In Vietnam, these strategies intersect with a governing apparatus in which state agents have long been charged with introducing government directives to citizens.

Social marketing originated in the United States during the First World War. It uses commercial marketing techniques to plan, execute, and evaluate programs that aim to influence the behavior of target audiences and thereby improve individual and social welfare. The social marketing approach to behavior change equates healthy behaviors with consumer products, and places the health "consumer" at the center of planning (Novelli 1990). In situations where healthy behaviors entail significant costs and negative connotations, social marketing employs qualitative research tools to elicit target consumers' perceptions, needs, and wants with regard to the desired behavior. One research tool is the focus group discussion, which identifies "motivations" and "barriers" to behavior change. Crucially, the marketing approach sees behavior change, not health, as the bottom line—the product to be sold. Critics therefore argue that social marketing follows a utilitarian ethical model that emphasizes ends over means, and manipulates individuals into certain behaviors regardless of their sociocultural effects (Buchanan, Reddy, and Hossain 1994).

Discomfort about the social marketing approach has led some health programmers to turn to development-oriented communications that promote "participatory" processes of social change. Within the participatory development framework, behavior changes are not predefined, but rather emerge naturally in conversations between health programmers and target communities. As one proponent of these communications approaches summarizes, "Community members rather than 'professionals' should be in charge of the [communications] decision and production processes" (Waisbord 2001, 20). Participatory health communications, then, is not only concerned with changing behaviors; it also tries to promote social capital and community advancement.

In Vietnam, these dual logics of health communication operate within a context of democratic centralism (*tập trung dân chủ*). Although the Communist Party cites Hồ Chí Minh's declaration "The people know, the people discuss, the people do, the people monitor" (*Dân biết, dân bàn, dân làm, dân kiểm tra*) to celebrate citizens' participation in socialist democracy, civic participation is in fact tightly controlled by the central government (Craig and

Porter 2006, 134–35). In democratic centralism, the ruling party organizes and mobilizes the population through a variety of instruments, including People's Committee offices and mass organizations, whose representatives instruct or train citizens on how to conduct themselves in accordance with state directives (Gainsborough 1997; Thayer 1992).[8] These arms of the state comprise the key instruments through which government agendas reach citizens.

Social marketing, participatory development, and socialist mass mobilization approaches intersected, and collided, in the behavior change interventions I observed. Within this landscape, BCC programmers negotiated often-incommensurable frames of reference, and experimented with new ways of governing populations. Michael Fischer calls such processes of negotiation and experimentation emergent forms of life, and suggests that ethnographers are uniquely privileged to watch the testing, demise, and survival of newly created social forms. Taking up Fischer's exhortation, I will now pry open the black box of BCC planning, wade through the powerful sentiments at play, and examine what ultimately counted as resources for bird flu governance (2005, 56–57).

THREE PRIORITY BEHAVIORS

When I arrived in Hanoi to conduct research on bird flu control, over a dozen BCC campaigns were being carried out across the country, and several NGOs asked me to assist them with their efforts. BCC programmers told me that they were keen to develop messages that were not only technically accurate but also culturally appropriate and motivational, and as such they hoped to gain insights from the visiting anthropologist. I found these statements curious. All the BCC campaigns I knew of employed Vietnamese health and development professionals, people who had much more firsthand experience in rural areas and among local communities than I did. But I also knew that in an arena of highly competitive HPAI programming, where NGOs and for-profits struggled to attract donor funding, having a foreign consultant with research skills, language, and some cultural know-how added legitimacy to interventions.

I agreed to take part in two behavior change campaigns, with the qualification that my participation would inform my own research on HPAI programming, and that I would be observing, documenting, and critiquing their activities. Here I limit my discussion to just one campaign, which I call the Three Priority Behaviors Campaign. This campaign proceeded from collaboration between a foreign for-profit organization, a humanitarian NGO, and district level veterinarians. As part of my participation, I helped develop focus group questionnaires, observed focus group discussions, joined programmers in conducting semi-structured interviews with farmers, attended workshops with local officials, and took part in strategizing meetings. Drawing on these experiences, here I focus on the processes through which health programmers developed BCC messages, rather than the ways that viewers received them. I do so because I want to examine the ideas and practices animating the communicative approach to managing population health. Although my focus on the programming side of BCC occludes its social impact and effects, it reveals the everyday negotiations through which new techniques of governance come to take shape in a historically and culturally specific health arena.

The Three Priority Behaviors campaign was funded by a multilateral donor and managed by a foreign for-profit development firm that partnered with an international nongovernmental organization and district veterinary agents. The donor is known for supporting international aid programs that promote market-driven development, which in the health sphere include privatizing health services and shifting health costs and responsibilities from governments to citizens (Buse and Walt 2002). In its HPAI activities, the donor operated within a framework of market competition, which meant that for-profit, non-profit, and nongovernmental agencies all competed for funding contracts to implement their bird flu programs. These agencies were also required to prove effective use of donor funds in order to secure future support. A for-profit research and consulting firm with no prior experience in Vietnam won the behavior change contract from the donor. This was significant because development projects in Vietnam are by and large carried out by nongovernmental and non-profit organizations. In contrast to these organizations, for-profit firms tend to be more concerned with measuring and quantifying the results, or success, of their interventions in order to appeal to funders *and* turn a profit (Keevers, Treleaven, and Sykes 2008). Keen to establish their reputation as a favored development organization in Vietnam, the firm's programmers aligned themselves with existing development interventions in the country, in which multinational organizations collaborate with state agencies to carry out projects. The firm chose to partner with an international humanitarian NGO with a strong reputation for its development work in Vietnam, and with veterinarians in the district People's Committee office where the campaign took place. In this partnership, the for-profit made all the strategic decisions regarding intervention financing, behavioral objectives, and key activities, while the NGO representatives and district veterinarians carried out the activities among target groups and relayed communications messages in face-to-face exchanges with citizens.

At the start of the intervention, the firm's project manager, Rebecca, asked

Cúc, one of her partners at the NGO, to develop a plan for on-the-ground communications activities. Cúc's first move was to consult a report on a participatory behavior change campaign that she had recently carried out for avian flu, in which villagers chose to adopt behaviors that corresponded to the specific needs of their communities. Cúc proudly showed me the report, which included glossy photographs of her moderating focus group discussions among commune leaders and villagers. The report's main finding was that BCC should "encourage people to use their existing knowledge and skills," and that "communication activities should be designed to be suitable to the community's 'taste' and [should be] created by local households themselves."

Cúc's emphasis on community members taking behavioral decisions did not sit well with the for-profit firm. Rebecca had hired an international behavior change consultant, Tarek, to review the NGO's proposed activities. In a written evaluation, Tarek criticized the NGO for inviting commune leaders and villagers to select certain behaviors according to the conditions in their communities. His report stated that such an approach

> [places local populations] in the role of communications experts, a role for which they may not be amply qualified. Similarly, delegating such critical tasks as drafting messages and designing support materials to commune level health and veterinary officials again assumes a level of expertise they may not possess, not to mention a loss of quality control.

Tarek recommended that programmers instead select a small number of target behaviors from the NSCAI's Gray Book, develop clear and concise messages that would motivate target audiences toward those behaviors, and repeat those messages over and over. "Say one thing, say it persuasively, say it again and again," was Tarek's mantra. His report included a series of text boxes marked with a bomb icon, which he used to dispel several apparently dangerous myths about behavior change. One read, "Myth: the local population knows best." His report further stated that allowing each commune to select its behavioral objectives would mean "a critical loss of uniformity in project strategy," both for the for-profit (which was piloting behavior change in three districts) and for the funder (which was looking to coordinate its health communications with NSCAI priorities).

Tarek's report points to a familiar argument between standardization and localization that continually gets played out in development programs and in market circumstances. The argument concerns the extent to which you can create a consumer product, or a development program, that caters to local tastes while at the same time packaging and distributing it *across* geographic and culturally specific settings. As I have shown, the diverse ecological settings and the heterogeneous exchange relations that characterize Vietnam's livestock economies belied efforts to implement standardized virus control measures, and designs to homogenize poultry markets and carry out mass inoculations failed to meet their targets. Standardization is tricky business in Vietnam's livestock economies.

And yet, from the for-profit's perspective standardization is crucial. This is because global health programming increasingly relies on evidence-based experimental interventions, whose outcomes must be measured and assessed. Tarek is therefore calling for the generation of reliable, comparable data to, in the words of the for-profit firm's website, "maximize the impact of donor assistance." Such data would justify scaling the interventions in the future (both in Vietnam and in other countries where the for-profit works, and where donor funds flow). The logic of creating standards to scale means that this behavior change experiment had to be deliberately disinterested in the specific biological and socioeconomic settings in which disease emergence and control took place. As the for-profit saw it, the aim of the behavior change campaign was to produce quality data and results for future funding and interventions, instead of nuanced understandings of local disease etiologies and local capacities for disease control. This is experimentality par excellence, a mode of governing that relies on intervention, and that obtains its legitimacy primarily from the data it produces, rather than its impact on health.

Following Tarek's advice, Rebecca decided that the campaign would promote three behaviors prioritized by the Gray Book: handwashing before and after contact with poultry; buying and selling healthy poultry; and reporting sick and dead poultry to veterinary officials. In making this choice, Rebecca was preoccupied with carrying out a campaign that catered to donor requirements to align behavioral messages with NSCAI priorities. This meant bypassing the more inductive and interactive processes of behavior change promoted by its partners at the humanitarian NGO. With the behavioral outcome of the intervention determined in advance, the process of engaging participants' input was not intended to learn about community aspirations or to engage communities in a productive dialogue about desired behaviors; rather, this process was meant to shape aspirations and induce desires.

Competition for donor funds also meant that programmers were preoccupied with demonstrating the success of the experiment even before it was initiated. Employees at the for-profit firm constantly discussed strategies for measuring the adoption of their three priority behaviors. In a meeting with representatives from their NGO partner, Tarek declared that it would be meaningless to promote behavior changes that could not be quantified to donors. In response, a rather shocked NGO partner replied, "But we have a moral obligation to promote behaviors that reduce the risk of disease!" Undeterred, Tarek countered, "There is a difference between risk perception and actual risks. There doesn't have to be a risk but people have to perceive a risk to change behavior." He described this task of creating risk perceptions as "winning the hearts and minds of target audiences," a hapless reference to American military strategies in Vietnam.

With this agenda in mind, programmers from the Three Priority Behaviors campaign worked to sell behaviors to citizens conceived of as health seeking consumers. As noted, the for-profit was working under a donor emphasis on health programming that reduces state funding and involvement in health services, and its objective was to engender a social movement to "build the capacity of communities to adopt healthier poultry keeping and consumption practices." In order to instill a sense of individual responsibility for community health, the for-profit adopted social marketing doctrines, and went to work on "persuasive and motivational messages to win over audiences." Tarek summed up the marketing strategy this way: "We've got to make bird flu sexy!"

Tarek and Rebecca started by proposing the use of focus groups to elicit the motivations and barriers to behavior change. They obtained focus group questionnaires developed by qualitative researchers at the for-profit's headquarters in the United States, and then handed them over to their partners at the NGO, Cúc and An. Cúc and An were both Vietnamese nationals who moderated the focus groups in target communities. Cúc was a medical doctor with extensive outreach experience in communities where the discussions took place. At the time of the intervention she was working both for the NGO and for the Vietnamese Ministry of Health, a joint appointment common to development work in Vietnam and standard practice in HPAI management. An was a social scientist who transited among different international NGOs in Vietnam conducting research for various development interventions. In addition to this pair, Đoàn, the district veterinarian in the target community, was tasked with populating the focus groups with the appropriate target audiences.

Given her experience with community based development work, Cúc was miffed that the for-profit had given her focus group questionnaires written by foreigners. The questionnaires were pages long and had many yes or no questions, for example: Do you wash you hands before and after contact with poultry? Why or why not? Do you think that washing your hands can prevent disease? Do you report dead poultry to your local vet? Why or why not?

Knowing that I was asked to report back to Rebecca on my impressions of the focus group discussions, Cúc told me that Rebecca's emphasis on getting too much information cut off meaningful engagement with the community. "How am I supposed to get through all of these questions in an hour? How are we supposed to have a discussion? They don't know the way of working in Vietnam. If I ask all of these questions, the people will think I am stupid!" Using development rhetoric of flexibility and local participation, she complained that the people were not talking openly, and that those writing the questions did not know what works in Vietnam. An agreed. He insisted that NGO workers have to instruct participants on how to answer the questions; otherwise they will answer yes to everything. Participatory health programming was a relatively new introduction to development work in Vietnam, and because of this An argued that citizens were not familiar with focus groups that encouraged them to state their opinions. From my own vantage point as an observer, the questions did seem to cut off opportunities for discussion, since participants were able to anticipate the "correct" answers to the questions (yes, of course we wash our hands after contact with poultry; yes, of course we notify vets if our animals get sick) and the questionnaires gave no instruction about where to go from there.

Cúc's frustration revealed more than the limits of the questionnaire, however. Employed simultaneously by the Vietnamese government and an international NGO, Cúc was not only acting in her capacity as a development worker, she was also approaching the focus group from her position as a medical doctor and government representative. As noted, Vietnam's socialist state planning mechanisms view the people as subjects to be instructed or led in correct ways by those higher in the governing hierarchy. Cúc was reluctant to ask questions that put her in a position of ignorance vis-à-vis villagers. Because of this positioning, and because the focus groups were getting very little information on citizens' actual health attitudes and practices, Cúc decided to instruct villagers on bird flu transmission routes and prevention techniques. She used an easel and paper to draw virus circulations within and across species lines, and answered questions about how long the pathogen could survive without a host. Cúc's improvisation turned out to be a problem for her collaborators. Instructing citizens on disease transmission was not the aim of the communications intervention, motivating behavior change was, and Rebecca told me that Cúc had a history of changing the questionnaires and "falling back on training." She added, "Sometimes we want their [NGO workers] input and sometimes we just want them to do what we tell them to."

And yet, Cúc's adherence to more directed, top-down forms of health communication resonated with those participating in the intervention. Once

the easel came out, focus group participants came alive. They actively listened and raised their hands for Cúc to clarify or expand on certain points.
At the end of nearly all of the focus group discussions, after dutifully answer-
ing questions and expressing a wish to learn more about HPAI, participants
broached the subject of funding. They asked Cúc to provide their commune
with funds to buy poultry antibiotics and vaccines, and to give them advice,
and money, to build hygienic poultry coops.[9] Of course, Cúc was unable to
provide these funds (the point of BCC is to cut expenses like these), but at
the end of the discussion each participant was given a small sum for taking
the time to join the focus group. Participants' reactions to training reflected
a long-standing form of political subjectivity in Vietnam, in which state representatives school citizens in appropriate conduct, and citizens in turn use
their role as subjects to their own ends.

The evolution of these focus group discussions reveals two important
points. First, in Vietnam neoliberal, cost-effective forms of health governance
are inflected by an ethos of social welfare in which authorities are expected
to train and support the people (Pashigian 2012, 546). Second, Vietnamese
health subjects interacted with new governing techniques by drawing on socialist logics of state-directed self-regulation.

BUYING INTO BEHAVIOR CHANGE

After gathering evidence from the focus groups, the for-profit firm assem-
bled a meeting with its NGO partners and district veterinarians to brain-
storm messaging materials for the three priority behaviors. Tarek began his
PowerPoint presentation by summarizing the social marketing model of behavior change communications. Behavior change messaging, he said, needs
to establish "brand appeal," by creating attractive products that encourage
communities to "buy in" to behavior change. Though it may seem curious,
even downright bizarre, to associate disease control with brand appeal, this
is an expression of health governance that uses discourses of freedom and
consumer choice as a means to shift responsibility for health care away from
the public sector. In his comprehensive examination of neoliberal health
communications, Mohan Dutta (2015) argues that the health commodity
approach is particularly popular in the Global South because it creates new
consumer desires through advertising, public relations campaigns, and the
individuation of risk. The development a health commodity market deflects
attention away from the deleterious processes of economic growth that have
impinged on livelihood strategies and created new health risks, while at the
same time maximizing profits for health organizations. And so while Tarek's

insistence on making bird flu sexy made many of his colleagues uncomfortable, it coincided well with the imperative to create a consumer base of at-risk individuals, and a corresponding market of healthy behaviors that placed the burden of disease control on their shoulders.

The conversation about branding centered on what kinds of materials should be developed to carry the behavioral messages, as well as the best "product placement" for such messages. Tarek began by offering, "Of course we need posters," since their images would "model the behaviors" visually for consumers. His colleague at the for-profit, a veterinarian and Vietnamese national, suggested stamping messages on the handheld fans that market vendors wave to keep flies from landing on meat products. Tarek thought this was a terrific idea, since livestock vendors come face-to-face with target audiences—direct to consumer advertising, as it were. Rebecca then suggested broadcasting a message over village loudspeakers. Introduced during the Second Indochina War, loudspeakers delivered news from the front and relayed motivational messages to maintain the war effort. Today, loudspeakers provide news on foreign and domestic politics, economics, and culture. Turning to her Vietnamese colleague, Rebecca asked, "Do villagers listen to those messages or do they ignore them?" Tarek said that it didn't matter whether people listened because the loudspeaker announcements were cheap and could reach mass audiences more efficiently than other merchandise. What's more, the number of listeners each loudspeaker reached could also be quantified. But Tarek wanted to make sure to include some sort of identifying jingle or tone to precede the announcement; brand recognition so that listeners could identify that the message came from the organization, and the funder.

Cúc then asked that the firm develop polo shirts for their veterinarian collaborators at the district level, which they could wear when interfacing with farmers. She noted that in a previous intervention, her NGO had given their outreach workers orange shirts with behavioral messages. Together, the garments' coloring and messaging advertised both the behavior and the NGO. Đoàn, the state veterinarian collaborator, was keen to get a shirt, but was quick to request white ones. Remember that white is the color of the laboratory tunics worn by state veterinarians as well as the scientists and professional veterinarians depicted in the propaganda images shared above. White is a color that implies knowledge and scientific authority, and sets health experts apart from health subjects.

Once they agreed upon the merchandising, Tarek spoke in greater detail about what messages to embrace and avoid. Some messages, he said, are stigmatizing and alienate audiences. Others are too negative. "Never develop a message that says, 'Don't do this, don't do that.'" Tarek's emphasis on positiv-

ity resonated well with socialist propaganda messages that used joyous images
of auspicious animals and smiling farmers to encourage particular production practices. These messages frequently start on a positive tone, deploying the Vietnamese term *hay*, meaning let's (as in, let's develop farming, let's
protect the family). Drawing a further connection to propaganda techniques,
he added, "You can also appeal to altruism" and show that the behavior is for
the good of the community. The appeal to altruism seemed to be the only
thing Tarek said that appealed to Cúc. She lit up at this point in the discussion: "The people will be happy to see that. Vietnamese people want to help
their community."

Community responsibility ended up figuring centrally in the resulting
behavioral messages developed by the for-profit firm. Fig. 14 shows one of
three posters issued by the intervention. Rebecca had hired an art agency in
Vietnam to create the posters, which had gone through several focus group
discussions to prove their marketability to rural dwellers. The image shown
image promotes the priority behavior of reporting disease outbreaks. It reads,
"Community health is a priority; notify veterinary authorities of sick or dead
poultry." In the image the farmer points to his healthy, active ducks and tells
his neighbor, "I always notify vets immediately if my chickens or ducks act
unusual." His companion answers, "If everyone were like you the whole
neighborhood would benefit." The farmer in this message takes personal responsibility, as well as responsibility for both his animals and his family, and
conducts himself accordingly. His wife in the background also conducts herself well, donning gloves, boots, and face mask on her way to their enclosed
chicken coop. In the image, the farmers act first and foremost for the health
of their household, which includes both flock and family, and then project
their care out to the community. The call for altruism is reinforced in the
logo at the bottom of the posters, which reads, "Care for poultry, a healthy
community."

The Three Priority Behaviors campaign also created a short TV spot to encourage healthy handwashing. The segment begins in the courtyard of a rural
household where three young children are playing a version of hopscotch. A
confident man enters the courtyard with a bag of goodies. The children are
ecstatic. They run around him, grabbing at his bag and shirt. Zoom in on
his face and you realize that the man is Xuân Bác, a well-known Vietnamese
actor and Goodwill ambassador. Smiling, he walks past the kids and glides
over to his sister, who is squatting above a newly slaughtered chicken. "You're
back," she announces happily. "I'm making you a chicken!"

Xuân Bác looks down and grimaces. A musical riff of The Who's "Won't
Get Fooled Again" signals that something is wrong. A pile of feathers is scat-

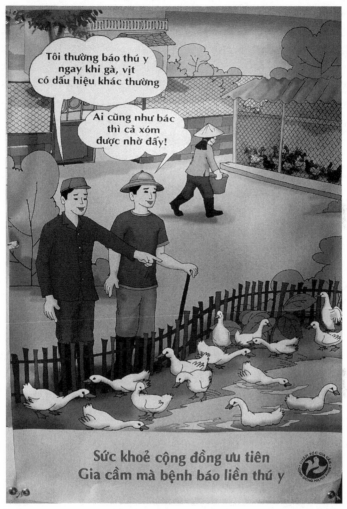

FIG. 14. Social marketing poster from the Three Priority Behaviors Campaign encouraging farmers to report poultry illness to local authorities. Photo by author.

tered around the water bin where his sister is rubbing the last plumes off of the chicken. She is squatting dangerously close to a rice bowl full of the blood recently eviscerated from the bird's neck. Gizzards lie on a chopping block nearby. Xuân Bác says in a resigned but caring tone, "Let me help you," and begins sawing the legs off of the bird. Together, they wash the animal and when they are finished his sister puts the body in a cooking pot and carries it away into the kitchen, walking directly over the feathers and blood before entering the house. Xuân Bác looks fondly at his sister but then glimpses the knife in his hand, which is covered in dried and caked blood. Crestfallen, he looks over the carnage on the ground. Innards and feathers and blood mix and mingle in the space between the children's play area and kitchen. He groans, shakes his head, and even sticks his tongue out when he realizes the enormity of the mess. He looks thoroughly out of place in this setting; his sparkling white sneakers, clean-pressed khaki pants, and crisp, *white* polo shirt reveal that he does not see much farm labor. Gingerly, he picks up the bowl of blood and disposes of the feathers.

His sister comes out and encourages him to leave everything alone. "I'll take care of it. Don't be in a hurry, come in and have some tea."

Younger brother is serious now. "All utensils must be cleaned immediately. There are a lot of bacteria in feathers, feces, and raw meat in general, such as avian influenza viruses and parasites. If waste is not managed and cleaned with soap, along with chopping boards, knives, and other things, they may spread and cause diseases."

His admiring sister looks into his eyes, "Now I know!" she says, and together the two lather everything in sight. Then, they wash their hands all the way up to their elbows.

"Done," Xuân Bác declares. "Now we can reduce health care costs by washing our hands with soap." His sister repeats the refrain. Then, he turns to address the audience; telling viewers that avian flu is a communicable disease and exhorting them to wash their hands clean of bacteria and viruses.

Though similar to the television spots described above, there are several distinguishing features of this behavior change message. First is the presence of the Vietnamese actor, whose name recognition was key to the firm's branding efforts. Second is the way in which the communications message belabored the handwashing activity, spending nearly thirty seconds zooming in on the siblings as they modeled the target behavior for audiences. It was not enough to relay information in this kind of messaging; knowledge exchange here required motivating audiences and giving them the necessary resources to adopt target behaviors. The segment also visually highlighted inappropriate hygiene activities, but overall the messaging stayed on point and positive as Xuân Bác imparted advice on the appropriate way to handle livestock. And finally, Xuân Bác uses technical terms to talk about viruses and bacteria, summoning science in a way that other HPAI messages do not, but that nevertheless resonate with patriotic hygiene campaigns of yore. His use of specialized terms positions him as an expert. This young man has all kinds of moral personhood. He is an educated man who has achieved fame, fortune, and success in a market economy, all while still expressing filial piety by caring for his less knowledgeable relatives back home.

In watching this video I am reminded of Cúc's interactions with farmers during focus group discussions. In this segment, Xuân Bác acted out a mode of engagement similar to her own, one that was respectful to farmers but also instructive. Health communication in this television spot hinged on training, but from a "cultured," family member, rather than a state agent. Top-down instruction was couched in a compelling image of familial responsibility, affect, and care. Xuân Bác's love for his older sister enabled him to sacrifice, or engage in activities he clearly found distasteful, and his superior scientific knowledge provoked him to instruct her in proper meat management. Neoliberalism's will to improve is evident (Li 2007, 5); Xuân Bác renders bird flu a technical problem that can be resolved through the application of scientific expertise and the enlightened reconfiguration of habits and desires. But he also renders bird flu a moral problem (Leshkowich 2012, 498), one that calls for the cultivation of proper personhood via proper social relations between fowl and family.

I want to spend a moment examining the gender dynamics in these BCC messages. The HPAI video clips shared in the previous section recapitulate the valorization of women's ability to solve social problems and uplift their loved ones. In the Three Priority Behaviors messages, however, we see virtuous men giving instruction on appropriate conduct. I want to suggest that this shift has to do with the politics of scale. Programmers were preoccupied with generating a social movement that sparked widespread behavioral changes. Each of the focus group discussions thus included individuals that local collaborators had identified as influencers and leaders in the communities. BCC programmers wanted to be sure that messaging would persuade them so that they could persuade others. In strategizing meetings, programmers agreed that these leaders would be men. And so even though there is much gender parity in government leadership and a long-standing valorization of women's productive labor in Vietnam, in this case we see how BCC posits other gendered ideas about who holds valuable scientific expertise, and who has the entrepreneurial chops to spread it.

Conclusion

Like model farms, vaccination, and market restrictions, behavior change communications constituted a novel, experimental health intervention. In the midst of uncertainty surrounding bird flu risks and the appropriate ways to manage it, HPAI programmers turned to communicative activities that encouraged bodily discipline and rationalized interspecies exchanges as a means to prevent infection. Behavior change communications was experimental on multiple fronts. First, it intervened on existing people-poultry-pathogen exchanges to engender an imagined future in which modern, rational health consumers took responsibility for their own well-being. Second, it brought different modes of governing populations together in novel ways, testing social marketing and participatory development frameworks in a socialist state context. Third, like the other experiments described in this book, BCC programmers generated new knowledge, monitoring and assessing their experiment's efficacy in situ, and as part of a broader program to scale interventions up and out.

Yet, even though BCC constituted an experiment in governing, its logics and practices were not wholly new or transformative. I have been at pains to show how so-called neoliberal governing measures like BCC have much in common with more sedimented forms of managing populations in Vietnam. To do so I compared mass media messages from the socialist period with those from the present era, and provided the historical and cultural context for understanding them. This mode of attention, at once genealogical and ethnographic,[10] allowed me to unearth continuities in governing techniques— namely, the rational application of science to solve problems associated with livestock development, and the leveraging of culturally specific virtues, namely sacrifice, as a means to improve the health and well-being of families, communities, and nation. Both forms of aesthetic governance economized life through the valorization of modern scientific sensibilities, while at the same time commoditizing life through the promotion of industrial, hygienic, and profitable livestock.

My analysis also unearthed some contestations and negotiations of governing strategies. In the Three Priority Behaviors campaign, participatory development frameworks that sought to bring citizens into the governing process met with various forms of top-down social mobilization—state agents instructing citizens on proper behavior, social marketers selling citizens on predefined behavioral commodities, and even citizens themselves expressing deep-seated modes of political subjectivity. These negotiations reveal the complex, multidirectional power dynamics operating in bird flu control, as state and nonstate agents vie for authority, and citizens make calculations on how best to navigate emergent governing regimes. Ultimately, the fact that Cúc's training techniques and other statist forms of didactic communication found expression in the BCC experiment reveals yet another continuity: both the self-responsible, socialist citizen and the self-responsible, neoliberal consumer have their options circumscribed, their choices limited by authorities. Self-regulation in a top-down fashion has a long genealogy in Vietnam.

Still, the extent to which any governing technique or authority can incite behavioral changes rests on its ability to leverage images and ideas that people find compelling. Calls for self-regulation and self-improvement have roots that reach further back than socialism, to Confucian moral codes that position the individual in extensive family and social networks. In Vietnam, self-responsibilization has always been a social endeavor. And so while educating and disciplining individuals to behave like model market actors may be a neoliberal idea, the fact that behavior change communications places individuals *in relation to others* shows that neoliberalism emerges within locally specific discourses and histories of control (Leshkowich 2012, 499).

Many scholars have questioned whether it makes sense to categorize the changes occurring in Asia over the last few decades as neoliberalism, and suggest that we would do better to ask how neoliberalism is established, especially in places with histories of socialism. Such an approach understands neoliberalism as contested, exceptional, and historically and culturally constituted (Kipnis 2007, 2008; Gainsborough 2010; Schwenkel and Leshkowich 2012; Ong 2006). Inspired by these scholars, I have used "neoliberal" as shorthand for governing techniques common to market capitalism—the conduct of conduct, the will to improve, and an audit culture fixated on assessment and results (Foucault 1991; Rose 2006; Li 2007; Strathern 2000). But I have also shown how such techniques were brought into conversation with other, sometimes strikingly similar approaches to governing in Vietnam. The dynamics of BCC programming described here show that "neoliberal," multinational organizations have not bulldozed the Vietnamese state; nor has the Vietnamese state bent multinational organizations to its will. Rather, the ideas, images, and techniques of behavior change reflect the enduring, yet shifting identity of the Vietnamese state and cultural values in global health.

How to Own a Virus

In 2015, health pundit Laurie Garrett published an opinion piece in *Foreign Policy News* exhorting the global public health system to do some "serious soul searching" in the aftermath of the worst Ebola crisis the world has ever seen. The bestselling author of *The Coming Plague* warned that, given how the crisis was handled, "it appears likely that no coherent scheme for saving lives in the next epidemic will emerge." Such incoherence, she argued, stems in part from a lack of clarity about how to handle virus samples:

> If the samples are removed from the countries, where should they go, and how can any decision be balanced against likely political outcry from the governments, neighboring African nations, and the world community as a whole? ... Who should now decide the fate of Ebola viruses stored in freezers in Liberia? How will profits be shared from products created based on viruses found in Sierra Leone? (Garrett 2015, "Ebola's Lessons").

In posing these questions, Garrett signaled tensions over virus sharing that have recently plagued pandemic surveillance and response activities. She also evoked a critical moment that brought these tensions to their tipping point. In 2006, the Indonesian government stopped sharing H5N1 samples with the WHO's global influenza surveillance network, which collects virus samples from around the world so that researchers can study emerging viruses and develop tools to address them. Indonesia's health minister at the time accused global pharmaceutical companies of profiting from vaccines and antivirals they developed from Indonesian flu viruses, all the while forsaking those most at risk for infection. In pointing out the simple irony that people disproportionately exposed to H5N1 were too poor to buy drugs to fight them, the Indonesian government alerted the world to the inherent inequalities of global health surveillance—that is, it politicized a process that was long considered apolitical: the effort to collect and repurpose viruses for the global public good. The outcry over virus sharing that ensued sparked four years of deliberation among WHO member states and drug developers, and culminated in a 2011 Pandemic Influenza Preparedness Framework (PIP) that acknowledged nations' sovereign rights over viruses found within their borders, and established new arrangements for more equitable virus exchange and benefit sharing (World Health Organization 2011). Nearly ten years on, Garrett wants to know whether Indonesia's claim of "viral sovereignty" (Holbrooke and Garrett 2008) will endure, and whether similar "special arrangements" will be made for other pathogens of pandemic potential.

Virus-sharing disputes reflect an experimental moment in global health. This is a moment marred by political and ethical debate, as schemes to protect global humanity intersect with agendas to safeguard national interests and efforts to promote corporate profit. Such debates are not new. Big Pharma has long been criticized for producing drugs that disadvantage the poor, and global health has long been plagued by questions about how to protect national populations and security interests. What are new, however, are the *journeys* that viruses take in an increasingly "data-centric" (Leonelli 2016) global health system, in which biological samples and the data derived from them travel the world at unprecedented rates. In this emerging sociotechnical arena, experiments in virus sharing intervene into the routine exchange relations that turn virus samples into data, knowledge, and marketable drugs; and in doing so they imagine a future in which vulnerable populations have more value in global health. Perhaps more than any other experiment in this book, virus sharing reveals how the commoditization of life forms (viruses) is inextricably intertwined with the economization of life, or the processes through which some lives are deemed more worthy of preservation than others.

I now take up an examination of virus sharing to better understand the relationship between life's economization and commoditization in global health. I am particularly concerned with virus sharing in One Health, which requires looking at the exchange of both human and nonhuman animal viruses. Carrying forward a multispecies perspective, I trace how human and avian H5N1 viruses move through globalized scientific institutions, data infrastructures, and pharmaceutical markets, and I expose curious disconnects in the journeys that these viruses take. Namely, I show that in spite of new arrangements for sharing human viruses, more conventional modes of sharing avian viruses persist. This is curious because, like their human counterparts, avian

H5N1 viruses are critical to global health activities: they are central to the identification of emerging pandemic strains; they are an essential resource for transnational research on zoonotic flu; and they comprise building blocks for pharmaceutical development. In short, avian viruses are valuable. Yet they have not attracted the kinds of ownership claims that could spark new and potentially more equitable arrangements in global health. Why?

I contend that if we look at the distinct biomedical and livestock economies in which human and avian viruses become commodities, we can better understand the differential articulation of value in One Health. I am thinking of value in the economic sense of how goods/commodities are measured and assessed in One Health, and in the sociological sense of what counts as good and desirable for those living under One Health governance—humans and animals included (Graeber 2001, 1). As I show below, nation-state claims over human viruses *tether* them to their human hosts and permit governments to make ethical arguments about the desire to preserve citizens' lives in the face of profit-driven pharmaceutical markets. These ethical arguments about the inherent value of life are harder to make, however, in the case of livestock. Livestock are disposable by design; their value is not inextricably tied to life, or health. What's more, livestock are commodities, not citizens. This means that any claims over livestock viruses fall *not* to nations, but rather to other actors who have different stakes in pandemic governance. The fact that flu viruses are tethered to livestock therefore upsets One Health efforts to unite human and animal health systems, and thwarts the ability of nation-states to assert their rights in global health orders.

Virus Surveillance and the Imperative to Share

Officially, human and animal influenza viruses travel in two separate yet interacting networks, each of which has its own institutions and histories of sharing. The human side of virus surveillance was established in 1952 and is currently called the Global Influenza Surveillance and Response System (GISRS). In this system, the WHO collects human virus samples from 113 participating nations and sends them onto certified laboratories for testing, genetic sequencing, and then further research and drug development. The animal side of virus surveillance was established in 2005 in response to H5N1. It's called OFFLU and is jointly coordinated by the World Organization for Animal Health (OIE) and the UN Food and Agricultural Organization (FAO). Like the WHO on the human side, the OIE/FAO collects animal virus samples from participating nations and sends them onto certified laboratories for research and drug development. Both networks genetically sequence viruses and publish that data so that scientists can look for troubling patterns and mutations.

Fig. 15 offers an ideal type rendering of human and animal virus movements within these networks. Their journey begins when human or animal health workers on the ground extract virus samples from infected subjects. The virus samples then travel to certified national laboratories that have passed either the WHO or OIE/FAO's external quality assessments. There, the samples are analyzed with real-time reverse-transcription polymerase chain reaction [RT-PCR] and deemed either positive or negative for H5N1. After that, the samples pass onto one of the thirteen WHO or nine OIE/FAO global reference laboratories to verify whether the virus is H5N1 positive or negative. After verifying the sample, the reference labs publish the virus's genetic sequence data on public databases such as FluNet (WHO), EMPRES (OIE/FAO), and/or the larger repository of genetic data, GenBank (National Institutes of Health). WHO and OIE/FAO officials insist that making sequence data publicly available is critical for a global One Health agenda that seeks to coordinate human and animal health, because it allows scientists on both sides of the species divide to stay abreast of strains that could potentially spill over and cause a pandemic.

Historically, these virus journeys have proceeded from an ethos of open source virus sample and data sharing (Fidler 2008).[1] Until recently, open sharing seemed obvious. Flu viruses evolve quickly, and so organizations like the WHO and OIE/FAO rely on the unencumbered exchange of virus samples to identify the most dangerous strains and to advise member states on critical life or death issues related to risk assessment, containment measures, and drug development. What's more, since the start of the new millennium, an Open Data movement in biology has seen scientists embracing the

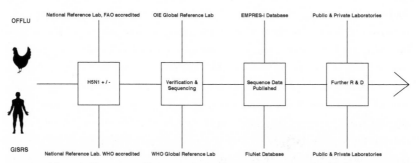

FIG. 15. Schematic illustration of human and animal virus sharing networks. The human network, GISRS, occupies the bottom half of the image while the animal network, OFFLU, takes up the top half. Image by author.

opportunities provided by digital technologies to circulate data in real time, no matter where they come from. Centralizing the collection of influenza data in repositories like FluNet, the argument goes, maximizes the chances of identifying significant mutations and patterns that can then be addressed in a timely manner. Open sharing, in other words, enhances scientists' ability to translate data into actionable knowledge (Leonelli 2016, 57).

It is in this work of turning data into actionable knowledge that virus sharing gets tricky, and where challenges to open source sharing start to emerge. Traditionally, after the virus sample has been characterized and its sequence information made available, the virus may go in one of several directions: it might be stored in a freezer or undergo further tests at the global reference lab, or it might move on to other private or public institutions for more research and/or pharmaceutical development. Along with the interpretation of sequence data, is through these movements that virus samples can come to take on added value—in scientific publications, funding schemes, and drug therapies. Depending upon the agreement worked out between laboratories, health officials and scientists from the virus-providing nation might *or might not* contribute to further research conducted on the virus sample, and they might *or might not* be privy to the knowledge such research generates. Perhaps most importantly, the virus-providing nation might *or might not* be in a position to directly benefit from that research, whether by obtaining drug therapies, contributing to scientific publications, or receiving public health applications. Given the ambivalence about the benefits that nations can accrue from open source exchange, the imperative to share underwent a profound disruption at the height of bird flu scares. It became experimental.

In 2006, amid fears that continued outbreaks of HPAI would lead to a human pandemic, the Indonesian government stopped forwarding human virus samples to the WHO. The health minister, Siti Fadilah Supari, justified this move by stating that the WHO was passing Indonesia's virus strains to an Australian pharmaceutical company (Commonwealth Serum Laboratories) without the government's consent, an act that violated WHO guidelines. Supari protested that this company used the strains to develop a patented vaccine that would be sold at prohibitive cost to Indonesia; this despite the fact that Indonesians are disproportionately at risk for infection (Supari 2008). In 2007, she stated, "Indonesia will insist on a material transfer agreement (MTA) before sending the Indonesian strain of bird flu virus to foreign laboratories to prevent them from being used for commercial purposes. . . . Until then, we won't share the samples" (Khor 2007). She also called for the closure of two US Naval Medical Research Units in Indonesia, arguing that Indonesian scientists and Indonesian laboratories should control H5N1 research.

To make its case, the Indonesian government cited rules on the protection of biological resources found in the 1992 UN Convention on Biological Diversity (CBD), which recognizes "the sovereign rights of States over their natural resources, the authority to determine access to genetic resources rests with the national governments and is subject to national legislation" (United Nations 1992, Article 15).[2] Prior to Indonesia's withholding of virus samples, however, the CBD had not been applied to viruses, in part because viruses have been understood as global threats in need of extermination rather than state resources in need of protection (Lakoff 2010, 62; Smallman 2013).[3]

Indonesia's decision to counter what it called "neocolonialism" in global health was unprecedented, and it split opinion within the international community. Policy makers and public health pundits criticized Indonesia's refusal to share virus samples as a reckless endangerment of global health security (Holbrooke and Garrett 2008). Galvanized by these admonishments, the former Indonesian ambassador to the United Nations stated that "viruses are, unequivocally, genetic resources subject to national sovereignty"(Wibisono 2008). Indonesia's claims were gaining traction. Soon after, authorities in India, Brazil, and Nigeria asserted rights over pathogens, and the Non-Aligned Movement of 112 developing nations formally considered the idea of claiming rights to viruses (Vezzani 2010).

Ultimately, Indonesia's actions sparked over four years of deliberation by WHO member states, which culminated in a landmark 2011 resolution that acknowledges a state's sovereign rights over biological resources, and encourages vaccine and antiviral developers to engage in contractual benefit-sharing arrangements with virus-supplying countries (through Standard Material Transfer Agreements, or SMTAs). Additionally, under PIP, virus-receiving nations now provide discretionary financial contributions to the virus-surveillance network, and the WHO has promised to distribute these funds to virus-providing nations, particularly "where pandemic preparedness is weak" (World Health Organization 2011, 6.14.9). Under the auspices of capacity building, these funds are slated for use in activities to strengthen state laboratories and surveillance, and in the training of domestic scientists.[4]

Tethering Life

Amy Hinterberger and I have argued that ownership claims in pandemic flu preparedness create *tethering* effects that anchor virus samples to specific territories and geopolitical bodies (Hinterberger and Porter 2015). The tethering effect of ownership claims has three key features. The first is territorial:

ownership claims tether biological materials to their territorial origins by delineating forms of specificity, or virus variation. Though they are not biologically confined to political boundaries, influenza viruses have long been specified territorially (for instance, Asian Flu and Spanish Flu, or in the country specific strains of H5N1 and H7N9). In drawing on the UN CBD, Siti Fadilah Supari asserted that virus strains form the biological patrimony of nations in which they are found (Smallman 2013, 25). Through this claim, she challenged a situation in which "poor countries have no bargaining power" over viruses, which traditionally acquire value only through sequencing or "human invented technologies," found in rich nations (Sedyaningsih et al. 2008, 487). In other words, tethering links virus variations to specific territories, populations, and bodies—prior to technoscientific interventions.

A second, related feature of the tethering effect is temporal: ownership claims tether biological materials in time, to the outbreak event, so as to harness their potential to become valuable as they move through biomedical markets. Turning viruses into useful research tools relies on technologies that add value through knowledge inputs, technical enhancements, or biological manipulation. Before a virus can be actionable for public health, it must be isolated from its biological milieu (host), its variations must be sequenced into data, and that data must be *interpreted*. Interpretation matters because not all viruses get picked up as relevant to global health concerns. Only certain strains will be developed into vaccines, and only certain strains will be identified up as having the potential to cause a pandemic. There is a lot of technoscientific work involved in assessing which viruses count—which viruses are good for pandemic governance. Interestingly, the unpredictability of what counts as "good data" (MacPhail 2014b) has created a situation in which money flows into data-centric biological research *before* data is interpreted and knowledge is produced. "Hype and hope" surrounds genetic data, creating promissory markets in which investors funnel money into research institutions with the expectation that they will see downstream returns (Fortun 2008; Sunder Rajan 2006). In other words, there is anticipatory value in virus research, which doesn't necessarily attach to any one data set or sample. As Frédéric Keck (2016) explains, collecting and storing virus samples in avian flu surveillance is both a technique of anticipation and a technique of collection, and identifying new and alarming viruses is only possible through the *accumulation* of both material and virtual information. More samples and sample data mean more potential value.

The promissory, anticipatory value of virus samples and genetic data is rearranging the temporalities of ownership in science. Traditionally, viruses cannot be owned until they have been transformed into genetic data and then interpreted by scientists, and researchers and biomedical commodity developers have relied on intellectual property (IP) to claim ownership over such added-value viruses. Several nations participating in the WHO's virus-sharing hearings, however, recognized the promissory value of viruses, and challenged IP frameworks by inserting claims earlier on in sharing arrangements. By tethering viruses to their geographic origin, ownership claims allow virus-proving nations to become value holders too, and this value adheres to the virus itself, in its material form. Tethering ascribes latent value to viruses at the outbreak event, when they are still in their "raw," material, un-sequenced state. Importantly, these ownership claims are not intellectual property claims; they do not transfer IP to virus samples. In fact, the PIP Framework includes a provision that prohibits virus providing or virus receiving nations to seek intellectual property on human biological specimens, virus isolates, or modified viruses (World Health Organization 2011, Article 6.1). Instead, claims over virus samples give nations bargaining rights in collaborative research networks regardless of their capacity to produce and interpret data or develop commodities—the traditional benchmarks of IP. Within the PIP framework, virus-sharing nations get financial incentives to share, access to vaccines and drugs, and inclusion in scientific research on virus samples and data (World Health Organization 2011, Articles 2, 4.A6). Locating value earlier on in the globalized research and development process thus allows affected nations to seek benefits from viruses even as they travel through space and time—as they move from laboratory to laboratory, as they transform from material to data, and then into evidentiary knowledge and, eventually, into public health applications like drug commodities.[5]

The third feature of the tethering effect is distributive, and is all about equality. Ownership claims disrupt imperatives to freely share biological samples for genetic research by highlighting how paradigms of open science continue to disadvantage those with less authority in global biomedicine.[6] Scholars have shown that the image of an open network forged on an equal plane does not capture emerging sovereign aggregates or centers of power in global health (Stephenson 2011, 628). Kaushik Sunder Rajan (2006) has described how biology surfaces differently in different national contexts, and that the promissory value of genetic research depends on older, often colonial, structures of inequality and subordination. It is no coincidence that Indonesia's health minister called virus-sharing arrangements neocolonial. Thailand's representative at the 2007 WHO hearings on virus sharing put it this way:

> We are sending our virus to the rich countries to produce antivirals and vac-
> cines. And when the pandemic occurs, they survive and we die. . . . We are not
> opposed to sharing . . . on the condition that every country will have equal
> opportunity to get access to vaccines and antivirals if such a pandemic occurs"
> (Branswell 2007, 05).

Claims over viruses, then, recognize the exclusionary potential of global biomedicine. They seek to transform exchange relations that espouse the value
of sharing and openness, but nevertheless reproduce inequalities between
populations and nations. In doing so, these claims challenge an economization of life that privileges those with more purchasing power in the global
economy.

Taken together, contestations over virus sharing forced the global health
community to admit that "sharing" should proceed in a more socially just
and equitable manner. A legal counsel for the WHO overseeing the PIP deliberations told me:

> What Indonesia did was wake us up to the fact that virus sharing is not just
> about surveillance. There has to be a response component as well. The key
> is equity. It showed developed countries that they are only as secure as their
> neighbors. Equity has a self-interest component and a solidarity component.

As a result of the deliberations on virus sharing, the WHO changed the nomenclature of the Global Influenza Surveillance Network (GISN) to the Global
Influenza Surveillance and Response System (GISRS). Virus-ownership
claims thus sparked new ways of organizing worldwide pandemic surveillance. Mobilizing notions of global equity and solidarity, the PIP framework
posits that it is no longer good enough to anticipate pandemics; the global
health community must also work together to *respond* to ongoing vulnerabilities in at-risk nations.

What's the Value of a Virus, Really? Or, Who are You Tethered To?

But before we celebrate this new paradigm of pandemic surveillance and response, we must first situate it within a One Health order that aims to bring
nonhuman animals into the fold of global public health. What I want to point
out here is that although the PIP framework has been hailed as a paradigm
shift in pandemic preparedness, its transformative potential so far remains
limited to the human side of virus sharing and surveillance. OFFLU, the animal flu surveillance network, has not yet witnessed moves toward the more
inclusive forms of virus ownership and benefit sharing seen in GISRS. Even
after the WHO deliberations concluded, OFFLU was slow to keep pace with

developments in human virus exchange. At an April 2011 meeting of OFFLU's Steering Committee, members noted the development of the PIP framework and responded by establishing their own working group to draft a "code of conduct" on sharing biological materials. Notably, OFFLU suggested that this code of conduct would act as *a stand-in* for the Standard Material Transfer Agreements (SMTAs) drafted by PIP.

OFFLU's move to bypass SMTAs is curious, given One Health efforts to streamline and harmonize the human and animal health sectors. In the human health arena, and in accordance with the PIP framework, SMTAs are critical for adjudicating virus sharing and for ensuring the equitable distribution of benefits to virus-providing nations. SMTAs delineate the financial contributions and drug-licensing agreements that virus-receiving nations and industries will provide to virus-providing nations, and they are the key mechanisms through which nations claim rights over human virus samples. Indeed, in the middle of the deliberations between Indonesia and the WHO, Siti Fadilah Supari stated, "Sharing must respect national laws, which means that Indonesia will be free to assert its rights over samples. The key outstanding concession Indonesia demands is that all shared virus samples be subject to a Material Transfer Agreement clearly setting out such rights." *Material Transfer Agreements* remind us that data comes from materials—from virus samples—which themselves come from somewhere.

OFFLU holds a different view on Material Transfer Agreements, which is published on its website:

> The conditions laid out in MTAs, together with the associated administrative burden, often lead to delays in exchange of material, which can impede diagnostic confirmation and/or further scientific research. Because the results of animal influenza diagnostic tests and research are considered global public goods, OIE and FAO recommend the rapid and effective exchange of material and dissemination of research findings (OFFLU 2018b, "Position").

In this statement, OFFLU places value on the "results" of material exchange: data and other research findings. In doing so, it pushes virus *materials* to the background of the research and development process. What's more, OFFLU defines research findings as "global public goods." This moralizing rhetoric elides the fact that findings come from somewhere. It deterritorializes the products of virus research and development, exhorts rapid sharing, and in doing so silences value claims that seek to address the unequal distribution of resources in pandemic flu governance. In this short statement, OFFLU essentially discounts what WHO member states took four years to recognize: in the geopolitics of global health, sequence information, research reports, diagnostic tools, vaccines, and drug therapies derived from virus samples are not global public goods, but rather are accessible to some and not others.[7] Such a retrogressive stance on virus sharing raises questions about what kind of public is being hailed in the "global public good."

It is perhaps not surprising that OFFLU has shied away from instigating changes to virus-sharing arrangements, since such transformations would overhaul existing exchange frameworks (after all, the PIP framework took four years to negotiate). What *is* surprising, though, is the fact that despite the precedent set by the PIP deliberations, affected countries have not agitated for different terms in animal virus sharing. I asked the legal counsel at the WHO who observed the PIP deliberations whether there were any moves to claim rights over nonhuman animal viruses. She said, "Right now there's no PIP equivalent in the animal health sector, but there is a lot of concern about it. The possible gains are huge for developing countries so it's something we're keeping our eye on, but so far nothing has come up." She intimated that a framework like PIP would be a reasonable development in the animal health sector, and that it could very plausibly emerge in the future. Why the delay?[8]

A year after the finalization of the PIP framework, I visited the UN FAO office in Hanoi to speak with a consultant on the global animal disease surveillance system (of which OFFLU is a part). He was in Vietnam to help train domestic animal health workers in avian flu surveillance activities. At my request, he walked me through the official surveillance process for avian H5N1 viruses in Vietnam:

> The exact procedures may vary, but the sample moves from the [regional] lab to the Department of Animal Health, to an OIE report, and then to one of the 9 global FAO/OIE Animal Health reference labs for verification. . . . The chain of movement and sample sharing varies country to country. There is no standard operating procedure. As far as "best practices" are concerned, there is a range of variability.

To learn more about the variable sample sharing activities on the ground, he suggested that I visit his colleague Lee. Lee was an FAO officer working at Hanoi's National Center for Veterinary Diagnostics, where he characterized virus samples from around the country and sent them onto global reference labs for further analysis. I made my way over to Lee's office at the northern outskirts of the city, where I met with him and his collaborator at the Vietnam Department of Animal Health (DAH), Bảo. I guessed that Lee was in his late forties, and judging by his locally purchased sandals, ruffled lab coat, and easy working relations with the staff mulling around the office, I surmised that he had been in the country for some time. Bảo was younger, with slicked-back hair, a crisp Oxford shirt, and an eager look in his eye. I was accustomed to this paired mode of interviewing, since in all avian flu–related activities foreign consultants worked alongside representatives from a corresponding government agency. Sometimes these partners presented a united front, with one doing the talking and the other inundating me with pamphlets, booklets, and handouts. Other times, in accordance with their particular organizational culture, one partner did all the talking. In rare instances the partners approached the interview as they would a conversation, and depending on their personalities and relationships, the discussion could get animated. This is what I experienced with Lee and Bảo.

I began the conversation by explaining my interest in virus-sharing practices for avian influenza. "I'm trying to trace how you actually transfer viruses between the DAH and FAO/OIE, and also between other labs for research and drug development."

Bảo responded quickly, and with some pride, "Oh, well we have 100 percent sharing with the CDC [U.S. Centers for Disease Control]."

This was not the response I expected. As I understood it, the CDC was a WHO reference lab, not an OIE/FAO reference lab. It lay in the *human* virus surveillance network. So I asked the pair why they sent the animal viruses to the CDC rather than to one of the labs in the OFFLU network. Bảo said, "Because those labs give poor feedback. When we sent samples to Geelong (the site of the Australian Animal Health Laboratory CISRO), we had to wait six months for results! And even then they only gave partial sequences that said yes, it's an H5 virus. We already knew that from the PCR! The CDC gives us results quickly, and they give us progress reports on the viruses."

Lee added, "The CDC also gives us reagents, and they publish with Vietnamese scientists. So we don't hesitate to send viruses to them. And the OIE labs only have animal viruses. The CDC has viruses from humans, mammals, and birds. Only they can do cross-species comparison work on all of these samples."

I asked, "So then does the DAH have a contract with the CDC when it sends the viruses?"

Lee turned to Bảo, "Are there Material Transfer Agreements?"

"I don't think so. We have a traditional relationship with the CDC."

"But what about the newcomers?" Lee asked. "The Japanese and Korean organizations? Do they have MTAs?"

"Not yet."

I prodded, "Well what do you do in the case of a private company, like a vaccine company?"

Bảo said, "For example, tomorrow I'm meeting with a French company for a dengue vaccine. But we don't sell them the virus; they don't have a right or an invoice. No cash."

Lee interjected, "But why not cash? A \$20,000 payment for the virus would not be a problem for these companies."

"The problem is we don't have a mechanism for it."

"So get a mechanism!"

"It has to go through the government."

"But are there any rules?"

"If it's good for Vietnam then we don't object."

"But what about financial profit?

"There aren't any previous examples!" Frazzled, Bảo picked up his phone, dialed a number, and continued. "Anyway, in the dengue case the Vietnam virus is a *human* one used for a vaccine candidate strain. These [animal] transactions are not well established." He then explained that he was inviting a colleague to join the conversation, a lawyer at the DAH who "knows all about the virus transfers."

I was rather startled by the direction Bảo and Lee's conversation was taking. These animal health specialists were unabashedly bypassing the animal flu surveillance network in favor of its human counterpart. What's more, Lee, an FAO representative, was openly criticizing the OIE, his organization's partner in One Health configurations of pandemic flu control. This was unusual. In my experience, health workers at both the national and supranational levels were very careful to praise the institutional collaborations stemming from H5N1, and only critiqued these arrangements after several conversations with me, and very seldom in front of their collaborators. Lee and Bảo, it seemed, had no qualms about pointing out the shortfalls of OFFLU, and they took advantage of the absence of standard operating procedures in animal virus sharing to forward their samples to laboratories that traffic in human and animal materials.

Like H5N1 viruses in the landscape, those circulating in technoscientific networks transcended species divisions. This was not an act of nature, but rather occurred because of unstandardized arrangements and ambiguous and unsatisfying exchanges among animal health laboratories. Lee and Bảo made deliberate decisions to share samples outside of the OFFLU laboratory network because they received things in return, data, reagents, publication opportunities, some of the very things that nations like Indonesia were asking for in the PIP deliberations. Far from codified, however, this sort of cross-species virus sharing relied on "traditional relationships" and localized decisions about what is "good for Vietnam."

The informal and even ad hoc nature of virus sharing became clearer to me once Bảo's colleague, Hoang, arrived. Bounding into the room from upstairs, Hoang patted Bảo on the shoulder, shook Lee's hand, and stood behind the two men, facing me. He smiled. Bảo told Hoang that we were discussing virus sharing.

I nodded and asked, "So when can we say the virus becomes proprietary? Who owns the virus?"

Lee sat back, "I never thought about it, you mean the virus or the information?"

"Well, that's part of the question. Both."

"Hmmm . . . actually the farmer should have ownership, and the virus goes through many people before it comes to us."

Bảo shook his head slightly, "When they make something. Modify it. That is the process."

"Well yeah," Lee agreed, "The person who isolates and analyzes the virus has ownership. But Bảo does a lot of publications on the virus and he always mentions in his acknowledgments the farm and farmers from where the virus came."

Bảo added, "I see IP as more technologies than materials used. IP comes when you can start to make money."

Hoang interrupted, "But the *virus* that the CDC keeps is the property of Vietnam, this is the agreement we have with them."

"But the CDC made a vaccine candidate virus using *reverse genetics*, and that's the property of the CDC," Lee argued.

"It depends upon the agreement," Hoang explained. "For these things the CDC will contact us and ask us for an agreement."

"Well, I think everything with the sharing should be dealt with common sense, and respect for each other. This drives the sharing."

Hoang pushed back, "No! There are MOUs [memorandums of under-standing]." He looked at me as if to clear up the confusion, "Listen, the regulations just aren't detailed or organized. They aren't well adapted to the biological sector. There is a policy but most labs don't know about it!"

"So the MOUs state exactly what the virus will be used for?" I asked.

"Yes, in the agreement it says, 'This virus will be used for this or that.' If they want to change the research, then they must notify the DAH. But there are still gray areas. Not all labs use the MOUs. Let's just say they're flexible."

Hoang turned to Lee, "I just met with [the EMPRES coordinator at the FAO], and he says that drawing up the MOUs will slow down the speed of sharing data. I said 'Come on! Our work is supported by the FAO!'"

Lee shot back, "Well, I work for the FAO, NCVD, *and* USAID. Everyone should be entitled to the information."

"But the work is the property of the Vietnamese government. The owner-ship is Vietnam!"

"Why is Vietnamese ownership important?" I asked Hoang.

"The main thing is we don't want Vietnam to be seen as just a worker, only sending viruses and not seeing what is inside. We want to improve own-ership by insisting that it's our property—they can work with us but it's our material."

I relay this conversation in detail because it encapsulates the sort of in-coherence that Garrett signals in virus sharing, and a lack of agreement on how to own, exchange, and value multispecies biomaterials. The Vietnamese example shows that in practice animal viruses can be claimed and leveraged for specific advantages, but *only when they jump species* to the human surveil-lance network. Even then it takes legwork and ad hoc agreements to recog-nize the ownership of animal samples. While the PIP framework has modi-fied a nation's rights over human viruses, Vietnam's animal viruses still come up against established IP frameworks that think about ownership in terms of knowledge products like scientific publications or commodities—that is, viruses with technoscientifically added value. In Bảo's words, property falls to technologies, not materials. Even though legal experts like Hoang embedded ownership in the virus samples, they confronted scientists loyal to these time-honored IP frameworks and the demands of officials who felt overburdened by MOUs and any claims that would impede data sharing. Against these obstacles, Hoang used Vietnamese law and legal channels to forge arrange-ments in which Vietnam is a collaborator, not just a supplier, in global virus exchange. In the absence of standard operating procedures, such agreements are experimental; they are negotiated amid a lot of "gray area," "flexibility," and, as the conversation makes clear, unknowns.

The experimental exchange relations coming out of Vietnam's animal health sector raise several questions: Where are the standard operating pro-cedures in OFFLU? Why is there a lack of clarity about MTAs and MOUs in the animal sector, especially in light of the precedent set by the WHO and GISRS? Why aren't state actors and institutions seeking more formal-ized rights over animal viruses, and instead leaving lawyers like Hoang to run around insisting that there *are* procedures for ownership?

The Speciation of Value

Tackling the question of why animal viruses have failed to attract systemic proprietary attachments requires taking a step back to examine the bodies and sites that these biomaterials are tethered to. In what follows, I consider the value that animal viruses generate as they move across different populations and territories, across different scientific institutions, and across different commodity markets. In doing so, I look for signs of tethering potential that could (1) impart value to viruses based on their territorial variations, (2) capitalize on viruses' promissory value in pharmaceutical markets, and (3) deploy virus sharing as leverage for achieving global health equity, namely through "capacity building" endeavors in affected countries.

THE RELATIVE VALUE OF VARIATION

I suggested above that tethering human viruses to nation-states capitalizes on the value of strain variations that emerge in particular populations and territories. The FAO consultant I spoke to in Hanoi emphasized the importance of eliciting site-specific virus variations:

> Sequencing is occurring more and more often now. Just a few years ago, it was much less frequent. This is due to a change in understandings of the value of sequence data. For example, sequencing shows that different virus clades can be found in different areas in the country and the Southeast Asian region, which could be better addressed through different, more targeted approaches based on the features of the clades.

To put it simply, regional variations in animal viruses are valuable for avian flu control. But for this specialist, such value lies in the sequence data, not the virus material or its territorial origins. He told me, "It's unclear when a virus becomes proprietary because sequence information increases the value of samples, and sequences get shared publicly in domains such as GenBank." For this One Health actor, ownership relies on adding value to biomaterials through technoscientific interventions that turn samples (materials) into sequences (data). This data-driven, value-added notion of biological ownership effectively uproots the virus from its temporal and territorial origins and replants it in a virtual space where value is aggregated and homogenous rather than embodied and specific. In 2008, the OIE adopted a resolution on the sharing of avian influenza viral material and information. It states, "*All information* about avian influenza viruses that can lead to the development of more effective prevention and control policies is a global public good and should be put into the public domain without delay" (International Committee of the OIE 2008, "Resolution"). Under the auspices of the global good, animal data repositories effectively sever the ties that would bind specific sequences to their material source, and thereby deny rights based on geographic specificity or biological patrimony.

As I noted above, this approach to eliciting, capturing, and de-territorializing viral variations was standard practice in both human and nonhuman animal virus surveillance prior to the PIP deliberations. It has a basis in biology, since the characteristics that impart value to virus strains also preclude their rootedness in place. Flu viruses are mutable *and mobile*. Variations only come to matter in pandemic preparedness because they do not respect the integrity of individual, species, or geopolitical bodies. H5N1 virus variants would not be valuable to *global* public health if they stayed in Indonesia. And indeed the biological dynamism of influenza viruses has led many detractors to argue that sovereignty is an inaccurate claim to make over such shifty entities.

But part of what makes viral sovereignty so effective in territorializing viruses is its ability to tether them to geographically situated and vulnerable *human populations*. There is a moral grounding to tethering, inasmuch as it focuses attention on what Aihwa Ong (2008) calls the sheer survival of national populations put at risk by particular pathogens. The moral grounds of survival, however, find little traction in situations where viruses infect livestock. To state the obvious, saving lives is not a primary goal of the poultry industry, and cost is a key factor determining whether virus sharing and surveillance will even be carried out in the event of a suspected outbreak. Livestock surveillance activities can follow their own internal trajectories, and there are multiple examples of outbreaks being handled entirely in-house (or on the farm), with farmers not reporting and/or quickly selling off sick birds, or by engaging in secretive mass slaughtering activities. Farmers (and consumers), in other words, are habituated to poultry death. It does not cause moral outrage. Further, from the perspective of farmers, while understanding the source of livestock death is important for maintaining productivity, knowing exactly which virus strain led to the loss of life is less important than knowing which measures to take to avoid infection and associated economic losses.

What's more, in places like Vietnam where avian flu is already enzootic (endemic to poultry), any number of avian flu virus variations can lead to the loss of poultry life (whereas so far only a select few variations can kill humans). Just as viruses become more valuable as they threaten to cross national borders, the most valuable viruses in One Health pandemic planning are those that have already transgressed the integrity of species boundaries. Put another way, the value of a human H5N1 virus to pandemic surveillance stems from its *rare* capacity to spill over, and the fact that it usually only infects one human body. Those avian flu viruses that circulate in animals are much more prolific, and their value to pandemic surveillance is much less certain. As the FAO surveillance consultant explained,

> one of five viruses found on a farm will be sequenced because chances are the virus will be the same for all five samples. Or if viruses are taken from outbreaks on farms in the same proximity, only one will be sequenced. This has to do with the costs of sequencing, but also has to do with the fact that it wouldn't make sense to sequence different viruses found under such circumstances, it would be redundant.

Remember that H5N1 viruses have infected hundreds of millions of domestic poultry and only a few hundred humans worldwide. The laws of supply and demand are in full effect in virus valuation.

THE RELATIVE VALUE OF PHARMACEUTICALS

If animal viruses find different value in surveillance activities, what of their worth to promissory pharmaceutical markets? The most important pharmaceutical intervention for avian H5N1 is vaccination. Recall that the equitable distribution of vaccines was at the very heart of the Indonesia's claims over virus samples. It stands to reason, then, that affected nations like Vietnam could use animal viruses as a lever to access poultry prophylactics. But animal vaccines circulate much differently than their human counterparts.[9] In a comprehensive review, Swayne and Spackman conclude that routine poultry vaccination only occurs in four countries: China, Egypt, Vietnam, and Indonesia. These enzootic nations (where H5N1 is endemic) comprise 99 percent of worldwide poultry vaccination, while other countries selectively utilize vaccines only after an outbreak or among high-risk populations. Only thirteen of sixty-nine countries affected by avian flu had poultry vaccine banks in 2010, and most did not indicate a desire to purchase more vaccines when their current stockpiles expired (2013, 79).

The low demand for poultry vaccines is tied to their dubious value as global public health interventions. Using vaccines to control the virus in animals has always been seen as a temporary, first step measure in staving off a human pandemic, and one that targets small- and medium-scale farms with less purchasing power than agro-industrial producers. When bird flu hit nations in Southeast Asia and elsewhere, many small farmers chose to stop production altogether rather than invest in measures to prevent outbreaks. This trend has increasingly left poultry production to the larger agro-industrial conglomerates that use a range of standardized biosecurity inputs and hygiene practices to prevent disease *in lieu of* vaccines.[10] Moreover, now that the disease is enzootic in poultry, with the H5N1 virus constantly mutating, the use of strain-specific poultry vaccines to prevent animal outbreaks has also come under question. In other words, in this bioeconomy, the value of animal virus variations is limited.

It is critical to remember that there are two markets at play with regards to poultry vaccination: biomedical and agricultural. Much of what makes poultry vaccination unappealing is the fact that inoculation negatively affects the value of poultry commodities in export markets. As Lee suggested, the owners of poultry viruses are actually farmers. But in the global livestock economy, vaccines can negatively impact farmers. H5N1 diagnostic tests cannot distinguish vaccinated from infected birds, and as such poultry importers do not accept products from vaccinated fowl. Livestock export markets have played a large role in vaccination decisions made by countries in Asia and Europe. For instance, Thailand, a country with world-ranking export trade in poultry meat, decided to "stamp out" H5N1 by rigorous surveillance, culling, and quarantine measures, and refrained from using any poultry vaccines. Further, even countries with national vaccination policies like Vietnam are preparing to enter poultry export markets, which would eventually prohibit the use of vaccination for disease control. Tethering viruses to their source in animals is arguably a less effective tool for obtaining benefits from biomedical markets. Poultry vaccines may not be a growth industry.[11]

THE RELATIVE VALUE OF CAPACITY

Vaccines were not the only "global health goods" under deliberation in the WHO hearings on virus sharing. Another key issue in the PIP deliberations was equity, which is frequently understood in terms of capacity building: making sure that affected nations have the resources in place to monitor and respond to virus outbreaks. In the human health sector, tethering biomaterials to their source has engendered new tools for bringing scientific research and development closer to the locations where it matters most. Recall that in the midst of the crisis over virus sharing, Fadilah Siti Supari called for the closure of two US Navy Army Medical Research Units so that domestic laboratories and domestic scientists could take control over pandemic flu research and development. And even though she criticized Indonesia's stance, Laurie Garrett and many other health pundits have also raised concerns about the availability of research institutions, laboratories, scientists, and first responders in pandemic-affected nations.

My experiences in Vietnam, however, suggest that capacity building takes on different meanings in different national contexts and economies. In interviews, Vietnamese virologists and state agents on both the human and animal health side did not seem to covet laboratory capacity to conduct advanced virological research. On the human health side, the head of virology at Vietnam's National Institute of Hygiene and Epidemiology told me, "Yes [the virus is] a natural resource of a country but if there is no capacity there is no value. Without a facility to learn about the virus there is no value. . . . Up to now Vietnam has not been concerned with developing a high biosecurity lab because maintaining it is difficult. Sharing activates the virus." Foreign consultants working in Vietnam were also less interested in opportunities to carry out cutting-edge research in-house. Lee reflected,

> We can't do much here; we do virus diagnosis and surveillance. Things like pathogenicity are out of Vietnam's capacity, so we are always looking for someone to answer these kinds of questions. To make a collaboration, that's good. . . . Vietnam's advantage is it has lots of biological materials and the field—the disease. Developed countries have the advanced technology and good facilities, but not the virus and disease, so it makes sense that we work together. . . . We can overcome financial difficulties by looking for collaborators. Our relationship with the CDC is a win/win. We get feedback on characteristics and sequences and they get the very, very valuable virus to keep.

Claims of virus ownership arise not only from national histories of inequality and exploitation, but also from national aspirations for collaboration and inclusion. In the Vietnamese national context, at least for these actors, virus sharing was not a leveraging tool for building capacity; it *was* capacity. Their views suggest that the measures articulated by PIP might not translate that well across nations that have their own peculiar political histories and agendas. Indonesia's claims over human viruses are rooted in a national context of anti-colonial activity, a growing biological conservation movement, and ongoing state appropriation of territory and natural resources (Tsing 2005; Lowe 2006; Li 2007, 2014). Although it inherits a similar history of anti-colonialism and state authoritarianism, in the last decade, at least officially, Vietnam has been increasingly open to foreign markets, investment, and policy influence. Bird flu in particular has been a key arena in which the government has made concerted efforts to attract multinational funding and partnerships. Vietnam is frequently celebrated by global health analysts for its open sharing of bird flu outbreak information and virus samples, and is often held up in contrast to secretive, inward-looking, and uncooperative nations like China and Indonesia (McKenna 2006).

Another issue complicating the relative value of capacity building is related to the ways in which the PIP Framework links capacity to nation-states and the rights and lives of their vulnerable citizens. As a UN organization, the WHO works within the structures and interests of nation-states, and PIP reflects that orientation. But livestock are not national citizens; they are commodities. Unlike humans, the vast majority of the world's poultry populations are distinguished by multinational brands, not national citizenship, which shifts the actors and institutions that can make proprietary claims over their viruses. Further, in much of the world, the best veterinary science is coming out of, or at least supported by, the private livestock sector, as major agro-industrial corporations outstrip public institutions in attracting talent and in carrying out research. Large poultry holders have their own networks of researchers with whom they share all kinds of samples, and they often fall outside of the purview of state and supranational public health authorities. In other words, these poultry corporations are resolutely multinational; they have even been characterized as a stateless oligarchy that prioritizes trade *secrets* rather than sharing.

Bringing national laboratories into the mix of livestock virus research would inevitably rub up against multinational corporations' interests in viruses, virus sequences, and virus therapies. And while Indonesia and others successfully bargained for new virus-sharing arrangements against Big Pharma, this is less likely to happen in the animal sector. Why? Because here the economization of life is different—and it goes hand in hand with life's commoditization. The fact that the poultry in question are already owned private commodities destined to die anyway weakens any ethical arguments that tie capacity building to public health and saving lives. In other words, when the aim is to commoditize livestock, rather than or in addition to protecting lives, private commercial actors bear more responsibility for disease control, and their interests gain precedence over those of public health.

Conclusion

The absence of synchronization in One Health virus-sharing and surveillance networks demonstrates that, for all the talk of species jumping and spillover, human and animal viruses live very different social lives. They travel through different bodies, different scientific institutions, different data infrastructures, and different commodity markets where they obtain very different sorts of value. Disconnects in how we value and traffic in viruses only begin to make sense when we situate these biomaterials in locally specific, multispecies exchange relations.

I have suggested that virus-sharing disputes reflect an experimental moment in global health. Claims of ownership over flu viruses are reorganizing political-economic relations between nation-states and corporate institutions, altering the exchange of resources in scientific research and development, and transforming the processes through which viruses become commodities. Flu surveillance has long rested on the idea that virus materials and data are global public goods that should be freely shared in the service of saving lives. Open source exchange reflects an understanding of viruses as a common threat rather than a national resource. It also reflects a deep-seated moral economy in the life sciences in which communities of researchers liberally exchange materials and information (Kohler 1994; Creager 2001). More recently, calls for open source exchange have been compounded by the development of new technical capacities that enable sequence data to travel through virtual networks where scientists can examine them in real time. Within these processes virus samples only begin to accrue value after techno-scientific manipulation, datafication, and interpretation.

Yet, even if we agree that the data circulating in open source databases have promissory value, there are several other points that cannot be denied. The first is that these data have more than scientific or even public health value. Biological data have political value as tools to legitimize governments, and as currency to be traded among national governments; they have financial value in generating downstream commodities like vaccines and antivirals; and they have social, affective, and moral value when attached to vulnerable bodies and populations (Leonelli 2016, 64). It is not good enough to limit the discussion of a virus's value to science or public health. The second point is that sequence data come from somewhere, from virus materials. This seemingly banal point is actually transformative, inasmuch as it allows virus-providing nations to tether viruses to their origins, and to seek benefits from the knowledge and products derived from them as they proceed along their journeys. Ultimately, virus-ownership claims expose the problems with a homogenizing and moralizing ideology of open source exchange — namely, that it erases the vital role that virus samples play in scientific research and national development, and occludes enduring geopolitical and institutional inequalities in global health.

But while the WHO has come to redress some of these problems through a recognition of virus ownership and sovereignty, its animal analog has yet to adopt a framework for equity, and there is a curious lack of agreement or standard operating procedure for avian H5N1 virus sharing. This is due in part to the fact that no nation has made explicit ownership claims over animal viruses. It is also due to the fact that OIE/FAO representatives resist the tools that would formalize processes for benefit sharing, like MTAs and MOUs, and instead suggest that, in the words of OFFLU's homepage, "scientists should rely on professionalism and trust when exchanging data and biological material to ensure that all contributors are acknowledged." Such commitments leave animal health workers and legal experts on the ground scrambling to claim virus ownership, whether by transcending species divides in sharing networks, or by establishing case by case agreements with laboratories and institutions. Without a mechanism or standard operating procedure to impart value on or ownership over virus samples, individuals like Hoang have to fight for national representation in increasingly global but persistently unequal networks of pandemic knowledge and resource exchange.

What I have suggested here is that the lack of codified claims over animal viruses in processes of biomedical research and commoditization may be related to an economization of life in One Health that values animals and humans differently. One of the arguments that social scientists have made about Indonesia's viral sovereignty case is that it inserts ethical considerations into the problem of virus sharing. Aihwa Ong (2008) suggests that biosovereignty creates a space of ethical exception, which focuses attention on the survival of human populations and challenges the power of global biocapital flows. Ownership claims work because they establish a bridge, or tether, between H5N1 viruses and vulnerable *humans* who have inherent moral worth in a global health regime that defines health as a basic human right. These exceptional claims buck human health and development interventions that have long privileged the lives of more effective market actors, namely, consumers with purchasing power. But animal viruses are primarily sourced from poultry; their worth is not given but rather surfaces in livestock economies where it is patently linked to death, not life. This calls into question any recourse to ethical claims about survival as a means to reconfigure exchange relations.

Such differential valuations of animal life find expression in One Health programs that posit animal slaughter as a key health intervention. In addition to the millions of animals that have died from H5N1 infections, even more have been purposefully destroyed to prevent transboundary disease spread. Those interventions that do safeguard poultry life do so as a means to protect humans or, more often, as a means to protect investments. Even in a One Health framework that seeks to integrate human and animal health, the loss of poultry to H5N1 is understood not so much as a public health problem as it is a livestock industry problem. The classification of poultry as both a life form and commodity permits its appraisal in regimes of value that operate according to quantifiable market metrics. This is not to say that economic losses are not important; indeed they have substantial influence on human livelihoods and health. However, such instrumental evaluations of poultry vitality do not lend themselves well to ethical claims about survival. Viruses are not the only life forms commoditized in livestock economies, and it turns out that H5N1 vaccines, the very life-saving commodities in question in the PIP deliberations, are worth much less in a nonhuman domain where value is attached to trade, not life. When the problem shifts from life to livestock, the modes of intervention and the ethical considerations attached to it also shift. Again, my point is not that human and animal lives should be valued equally in One Health (though that is a point worth considering). Rather, I am suggesting that the differential valuations of these life forms have all sorts of cascading effects on the kinds of bargaining power and rights that farmers, scientists, and nations can have in globalized One Health orders. These effects matter, if we are to avoid recapitulating the inequalities that continue to plague global health.

Virus sharing is an emergent form of life. The rules, habits, customs, and examples that guide behavior are in flux, and different actors are negotiating these contingent social arrangements in transformative ways. Life forms are gaining more and more importance in these negotiations. Claims of ownership demonstrate how viruses, as quasi-living microbial agents, come to matter in One Health. *But they matter differently.* In order to understand the range of experimental exchanges taking place in virus sharing, it is critical to understand the different contours and stakes of human-microbe and avian-microbe relationships. Anthropologists have begun to take microbes seriously in analyses of social and cultural life, examining the roles that particular pathogens play in food politics, infectious disease, and scientific knowledge production (Benezra 2016; Dunn 2005; Helmreich 2009; Koch 2013; Lorimer 2018; Nading 2016; Paxson 2008). Central to these investigations are questions about how scientists and lay communities understand and experience microbes (viral and otherwise), and how they use microbial data to intervene on health. Crucially, this scholarship can have a practical orientation, pushing for more accountable, ethical, and effective scientific practices (Benezra 2017). Here I have argued that microbial relations are species-specific. The biological, political, and moral stakes of human-virus and avian-virus relations differ markedly, and these differences have everything to do with the economies in which microbial relations emerge. If One Health is to engage in more ethical and effective forms of virus sharing and governance, its practitioners will have to pay better attention to these economies and how they economize and commoditize different life forms. Doing so will reveal some hard truths about the feasibility of harmonizing human and nonhuman animal health. It may even provoke a serious reconsideration of the idea that there is, or can be, "One" Health in multispecies worlds.

Conclusion

"All lives have equal value."

These are the words that greet visitors to the website for the Bill and Melinda Gates Foundation, the world's largest private organization working to improve health care around the globe. Arranged in a simple statement, they encapsulate the rhetoric of equality and concern for the common good that pervade global health. The World Health Organization website adopts this rhetoric in its mission statement, "to ensure the highest attainable level of health for all people." The World Organization for Animal Health does the same, but in a more expansive, One Health mission that addresses the "risks for human and animal health and ecosystem health as a whole."

These are powerful proclamations, and yet in practice global health and its One Health variant inevitably value different lives differently. On the surface this is not a particularly innovative insight; countless studies have shown the uneven effects of global health interventions worldwide. But I contend that it is critical to understand precisely *how* One Health values and intervenes upon different lives and ways of living with others differently, and how it does so within particular political, economic, social, and epidemiological contexts. Such an understanding is critical because it exposes a nascent One Health order that, for all its talk of the common good, proceeds according to economic principles of market competition and species standardization— principles that belie any claim to valuing lives equally, as well as any claim that One Health is just about health.

In this book I have theorized One Health governance through an ethnographic examination of experimental multispecies exchange relations. I started with a question about how bird flu control programs bring humans and nonhumans into the fold of a One Health agenda, and I proposed to examine what this process looks like in livestock economies where different life forms and forms of life intersect and collide. I proceeded from the notion that people, poultry, and pathogens create social worlds together, by engaging in meaningful relationships at a variety of sites and scales. What my analysis has shown is that, at every level and in every relation, some lives matter more than others. At the same time, these multispecies relations are unstable; they shift and morph over the course of health interventions as different actors and entities negotiate their place in Vietnam's changing livestock economy. Further, as the relations change, so do health interventions. Bird flu interventions are experimental. They apply inconclusive scientific and social scientific knowledge to disease-control activities, and they generate more knowledge through the process of intervening. In a context of ongoing avian flu outbreaks, a growing agenda to integrate human and animal health systems worldwide, and unclear evidence about the efficacy of any one strategy to stem HPAI, One Health interventions try out and tinker with various strategies to forestall the coming plague. Each of these strategies has its own objectives and imagined futures, but all of them have consequences for the different groups of human and nonhuman animals living together in Vietnam.

I conclude by bringing these two insights together: an ethnographic schematic of the experimental, multispecies exchange relations that shape One Health governance, and a consideration of how these relations privilege certain futures in which only some life forms and forms of life have value. In doing so, I propose opening One Health up to new experimental designs, which can better reflect multiple ways of classifying, controlling, and valuing life, and can better accommodate multiple ways of living with others in a pandemic age.

More-than-Human Health

To understand the stakes and implications of One Health governance, it is imperative to record how bird flu outbreaks and their related control programs generate *species-specific* effects. I start with viruses, microbes that not only lie at the heart of bird flu outbreaks, but also form part of the social fabric. Bird flu outbreaks provide viruses with opportunities to expand the range of hosts and ecologies in which to replicate, evolve, and flourish. Dropping from the feces of a wild bird into a chicken flock, for instance, enables contact with new, domesticated avian hosts, which (if they don't die first) could foster further contact with a pig, a poultry farmer, a neighbor, a family member, or even a motorbike or other infectious surface. If it is warm and wet enough, and the host moves fast enough, viruses can spread into a nearby market where opportunities to infect other living creatures and environments multiply. Viruses and their offspring could infect a vendor or consumer, other livestock, or perhaps an exotic creature for sale. From there they could spread in a number of productive directions, adapting to different host immunities and habitats, and transforming into stronger, more productive, more transmissible, and more or less lethal agents.

But alongside outbreaks come control measures with altogether different effects on viruses. The introduction of material technologies like vaccines and antivirals, fences and footbaths, soap and protective gear can kill viruses on contact, or later on by preventing entry into a host that has not yet succumbed to infection. Culls, quarantines, and agricultural zoning measures may also decimate entire virus strains, or isolate them in time and space so that they will perish before they are able to find new immune systems to exploit. But not all hope is lost for the virus, for even if targeted control measures like vaccines obstruct virus strains in the here and now, they create the conditions for new strains to evolve and reemerge later on and in more hospitable bodies and environments.

Some control measures deliberately extend a virus's longevity, though in rather less familiar circumstances. Global influenza surveillance systems sample, sequence, and stockpile flu viruses, effectively immortalizing them as material substances and virtual data for ongoing research and pharmaceutical production. This is a value chain with much potential for viruses, for even if it prevents them from propagating "in the wild," research and development all but ensure their replication and continued survival in the lab, in reports, in databases, and in promissory drug markets. Viruses, then, are not just disease-causing agents. They circulate within different epidemiological, political-economic, and sociocultural domains, mobilizing unique management strategies, forms of expertise, and objectives along the way.

A bird flu outbreak is an altogether different experience for livestock. Chickens, at least in their current form, do not stand much of a chance against H5N1 viruses; and this goes not only for those directly infected, but also for those in close proximity. There are a few potential outcomes for chickens in an outbreak scenario: they might become ill and die within a few hours or days, infecting their fellow fowl along the way. Another possibility is that their farmer-caretaker detects the illness early on and expediently kills the chicken and the entire flock, cutting his losses by selling the flesh to unsuspecting consumers. Or, the farmer may report the illness to veterinary authorities. This too results in death; vets will not only kill the infected fowl and their flock mates, but also all of the other poultry flocks within a predetermined radius. In this case, chickens will end up in a pit of corpses disintegrated by fire and lye. For their part, ducks may fare somewhat better. These "silent reservoirs" can sometimes carry the virus without displaying symptoms, thereby avoiding the terrible responses to flu so commonly seen in chickens. But ducks can still get sick and die from a bird flu virus, and the likelihood of infection may be somewhat elevated since in Vietnam ducks enjoy more freedom of movement and therefore more potential contact with wild (particularly water) birds—the virus's native hosts. Of course, livestock ducks and chickens are destined to die regardless of whether they become infected with flu or not. But with H5N1, their death will be premature, and it will lack the meaning and value that comes along with a planned demise. Livestock's status as a form of capital does not negate the important role these animals play in social life and in historical and cultural processes of identity formation.

Virus control measures bring both chickens and ducks into exchange relations with new actors and ecologies. The material technologies that target the flu virus largely do so while it resides in its avian host. For poultry in flu-affected countries, this means being handled, inspected, sampled, and probed in multiple ways and multiple times over the life course. The manipulation of poultry bodies and biological processes is certainly not new to poultry, but in the context of One Health these bodily interventions are carried out by actors with whom they have not had previous contact: agricultural extension workers, mass organization members, public and private veterinarians, and foreign consultants. What's more, poultry's living conditions may change. Farm restructuring interventions may confine them to limited holdings, or expand their dwellings by removing them from the environments they once knew. Poultry must therefore learn to socialize and make place in foreign territories. At the same time, they may also be subjected to new productive regimens that, while meant to protect them, could also make them sick and/ or expose them to other threats, including vaccine resistant flu strains or antimicrobial resistant pathogens.

But bird flu governance provides new opportunities for poultry as well. Industrialized, commercial brands in particular are seeing new avenues to expand their presence in Vietnamese markets, especially in urban areas where commercial value chains are making headway. Whether or not Vietnamese poultry will eventually transcend national borders and become a viable global commodity is yet to be determined, but their chances will be better if the birds can withstand standardized biosecure production practices while at the same time keeping the price of their upkeep down and their market value up. Local breeds, on the other hand, may be phased out, they may go underground, or they may be crossbred with commercial varieties for entry into niche markets that merge tradition and technique in novel ways. Whatever path local breeds take, their days of dominating the domestic market are dwindling. Livestock production, after all, is never innocent; it is rife with the displacement and dispossession (Franklin 2007).

For farmers, too, bird flu signals both peril and possibility. The unluckiest among them could contract the virus through contact with infectious fowl or other livestock. If this happens, the chances of recovery are slim. But farmers can take heart in the fact that they are unlikely to spread the virus to other people. Now, if a farmer escapes illness but their flock gets infected, then they could try and sell the birds as meat, or they could notify the authorities. In both cases, all of their birds will die prematurely. Farmers can recuperate some financial losses through the preemptory sale of birds, or via the compensatory mechanism available in their specific province. But they must be ready to take a large financial hit in either case. If they are among the few that have enough saved, then they may be able to replace the flock, but only after a period of disinfection and quarantine that suspends their earning potential. There are social effects, too, because if the farmers' neighbors' flocks are culled as a preventative measure, and if local markets depress as a result of bad publicity surrounding the outbreak, then the farmer with the infected flock can expect resentment to accompany any sympathy for their loss. If enough of these biological and socioeconomic costs add up, some farmers may decide to remove themselves from poultry production altogether and concentrate on other livelihood strategies, though most of these require financial investments that they may not be able to afford.

HPAI control measures favor the more affluent and entrepreneurial farmers. Those willing to dip into savings and/or take out a loan from relatives or state banks have adopted the biosecure breeds and production standards that allow them to propel their business into new commercial value chains and markets. However, such a move often means relocating to biosecure production zones and away from natal villages and familial rice paddies. It also means that production standards, trading partners, and prices are determined by an outside entity, whether a commercial or state poultry holding, or a nongovernmental organization. The loss of autonomy here should not be underestimated, as independent poultry production has long been a strategy for rural dwellers to cope with misguided agricultural governance policies. Independent poultry production has also engendered meaningful social arenas that tie farmers, fowl, and family members together in embodied relationships of mutual dependence, obligation, and care. The ties that bind are not so easily broken by principles of market competition and species standardization. In other words, bird flu creates opportunities, but these opportunities are both conditioned by and poised to recapitulate existing socioeconomic inequalities and problematic patterns of agricultural governance in Vietnam.

Of course, outbreaks do not just affect farmers and fowl. Health workers, too, bear the burden of bird flu. State veterinarians in particular stand to gain or lose a lot in the event of an outbreak. In a Vietnamese health arena increasingly fixated on counting and enumeration, when a flock falls ill in a vet's jurisdiction, he or she may be fined or otherwise held responsible. Vets also have to carry out a variety of new bird flu preparedness and preventative measures in addition to all of the other livestock-related activities they already engage in. They must be prepared to participate in market and farm surveillance activities at least once a week, where they probe and prod fowl for blood samples and in turn raise the ire of farmers and vendors for whom the detection of virus means the loss of income. They must also be prepared to spend days at a time in tedious avian flu training workshops, where outsiders (foreign health specialists and urban development workers who often seem spectacularly naive about local livestock economies) tell them not only how to fight against the virus, but also how to discourage the unhealthy habits of neighbors and friends, as if those actions are socially inconsequential.

Finally, vets must be prepared to engage in mass vaccination: the once short-term but now protracted first line defense against bird flu. In the best case scenarios vets can get farmers in their jurisdiction to agree to vaccinate, and somehow manage to secure enough vaccine for the task. But it is not uncommon to fall short, which means incomplete vaccination, farmer dissatisfaction, and a higher risk of infection. And even if there is enough vaccine and farmer participation, this does not mean that vets have the human resources to get the job done in what are often inhospitable ecologies and hard to access poultry holdings. Vets may therefore have to partner with semi-trained, seasonal veterinarians whose lack of experience and commitment to the work do little to raise their already feeble standing in many farmers' eyes.

Still, the presence of veterinary para-professionals in livestock economies demonstrates the potential gains to be made from this pharmaceutical intervention, since vets may be able to charge a small fee (monetary or otherwise) for such services. Veterinarians with access to commodities associated with livestock can and do exploit the new market for vaccines by engaging in private transactions. But this is a double-edged sword. Even if vets do not engage in side operations, or even if they come by their inoculations honestly, some farmers may accuse them of taking state-subsidized vaccine and turning them into personal profits.

State leaders face arguably even greater risks and responsibilities. Government officials and other policy makers are acting within a geopolitical field in which global health threats like bird flu compromise national security and sovereignty. These individuals must decide quickly whether to report new outbreaks, not only to citizens, but also to the World Health Organization. Vietnamese officials work in a middle-income country with a marked decline in state-provided health services, and a concomitant desire to participate in transnational partnerships and markets. Such conditions have prompted them to cooperate with the global One Health apparatus and report the presence of virus. Reporting has brought human, financial, and technical resources into the country to combat the disease; but along with these resources has come a host of new responsibilities. Officials face the bureaucratic and technical nightmare of establishing networked surveillance systems, functional laboratory diagnostics and biosafety measures, infection control guidelines in hospitals and other medical centers, outbreak response protocols, biosecurity targets in markets and farms, and a coordination mechanism for the myriad multinational funds, agents, and activities funneling into the country.

Bird flu also projects officials into a space of governance where nonstate organizations may assume some roles of the nation-state, and with a degree of autonomy from government bodies. The presence of non-profit, for-profit, and humanitarian organizations offering avenues to health care may complicate citizens' expectations of state patronage and stewardship, and give rise to some uncertainty about who to turn to, not only in the event of an emergency but also for everyday health issues. It is the government official's task is to figure out how best to integrate these global health agencies and bodies into state infrastructures, processes, and resource flows, providing them with a level of autonomy while at the same time making sure they are held accountable to domestic concerns.

Officials must also anticipate market shocks, declines in foreign investment, lags in tourism, and bad publicity. They must proceed with resolve, and caution, to avoid panic and further losses. Officials have taken the best of Vietnam's socialist state apparatus and combined it with a demonstration of the government's willingness to engage with multinational global health authorities. Namely, they have established mandates and collaboration mechanisms to ensure state presence in decisions and activities surrounding disease control and prevention, and they have leveraged resources, human and otherwise, to bolster state institutions in preparation for the day when global goodwill inevitably runs out.

In addition to all of this institutional and geopolitical maneuvering, officials face the broader task of safeguarding Vietnam's human and non-human animal populations. Their responses to bird flu outbreaks must therefore weigh multiple lives and livelihood strategies against one another. With limited resources they must decide, without definitive evidence, whether it is the household or commercial poultry farm that is most at risk for virus infection, taking into account which production system is more likely to promote the long-term health of the country's domestic livestock economy. Decisions about how to economize life are shaping the futures of the vast majority of Vietnam's citizens who depend upon poultry keeping for part or all of their income. Protecting the population at large from pathogens has meant launching many individuals into (further) poverty. This is to say nothing of the millions of poultry whose lives and life courses are impacted by official responses to outbreaks. Entire poultry varieties and farming systems have come under threat as a result of the decisions officials have made about desirable poultry commodity chains.

There are also opportunities to be had. Cooperating with the global health apparatus has increased Vietnam's international standing and generated new investments and partnerships. Vietnamese officials have also shown that by aligning disease control with agro-industrial poultry production, they can funnel transnational health resources into the modernization and rationalization of the domestic livestock economy. Bird flu policies thus continue a state-driven process of livestock rationalization that began decades earlier, during the revolutionary period. This will devastate many small farmers, but it could also improve the country's GDP. Further, state officials have taken advantage of the new conduits for multinational partnerships popping up around bird flu. Such partnerships have bolstered state health institutions while reducing costs, thereby facilitating Vietnam's market transition while maintaining state presence in citizens' everyday lives. In these "para-statal" partnerships (Geissler 2015), even if the state is not fully in control of health policy and provision, it remains tangible in health workforces and procedures, as well as in citizens' expectation of care (see also Pashigian 2012).

Finally, for those employed by one of the many institutions within the multinational global health apparatus, there are costs and responsibilities too. Multinational health workers' task is to prevent the next pandemic, which means that their responsibility is nominally to the whole of humanity—that is, the common good that animates global health (Montoya 2012). If they work within one of the global health institutions that proceed from a One Health agenda, their responsibility goes even further, transcending humans to include other animals and the environment. But while their orientation is global in scope, their individual labor is likely to be more local and discrete. Harmonization and coordination are the name of the game in the multinational health sector, for whatever the objective of any one intervention, foreign health workers have to establish relationships with the myriad actors and agencies assembling around bird flu in Vietnam. They must link up with other nongovernmental, multilateral, and multinational entities by sharing expertise, data, resources, and personnel. The most successful multinational health workers find collaborators among the cadre of government agents assigned to work on bird flu, because in Vietnam's health and development sector, nongovernmental organizations inevitably crisscross, act in parallel, and touch up with state institutions and structures. In addition to forming partnerships with government agents, multinational health workers must also encourage "buy in" from the targets of their interventions, which means courting the participation and conducting the conduct of farmers and fowl.

But even in spite of moves to create harmony and coordination within the multinational bird flu apparatus, global health workers are also enrolled in a space of competition for funds, experts, and other resources. They must therefore take the long view and develop and execute governing measures with an eye toward demonstrating efficacy, less to everyday citizens and local officials than to foreign donors. Those developing interventions therefore have to consider whether they can quantify their success, in samples collected, vaccines distributed, populations reached, or lessons learned. This might mean shifting objectives from saving lives to more measurable outcomes that can better justify their intervention's costs. Those interventions that successfully quantify their "success" can be scaled up in future interventions for future outbreaks in far-flung areas, creating new opportunities for health workers to continue on in their careers.

And so it goes. The diverse actors enrolled in the everyday work of bird flu governance navigate an emergent social arena with multiple different, intersecting interests, and not much agreement about how to proceed. At play in this emergent arena are differences between human and nonhuman animal health agendas; differences between socialist and market-oriented forms of governance; differences between local, state and global institutions; and differences between scientific, commercial, and other forms of cultural value. All of the actors and entities affected by bird flu navigate these differences, and they take the unique risks and opportunities presented by bird flu and try to translate them into value. I have argued that this work, of translating bird flu into value, is experimental.

Experimental Value(s)

Bird flu interventions take place on rice farms and delta paddies, in markets and homes, and along interconnected roadways, laboratories, and virtual networks. These are not enclosed environments whose conditions can be controlled or even fully accounted for. Interventions also bring together different ideas and agendas: they promote poultry production while preventing infection; they empower farmers while changing their behaviors; they increase veterinary capacity while vaccinating poultry. In other words, bird flu interventions bring public health systems and livestock economies into relation, and in ways that fuse *and confuse* economic, epidemiological, and ethical considerations.

Throughout this book, I have understood bird flu interventions as experimental systems that draw together different ideas, practices, objectives, and organisms; and I have adopted an ethnographic approach that traces how different entities react to experimental conditions in ways that cannot always be anticipated or accounted for (Rheinberger 1997). The concept of experimental systems helps me think through bird flu interventions for several reasons. First, these interventions take place in situations of unprecedented poultry deaths and epidemiological uncertainty, and as such notions of urgency and emergency fuel a moral desire to act even in the absence of validated scientific knowledge. This means that interventions often proceed without a clear question or theory to test, acting first and then observing what happens, even changing course along the way to generate better results. If we look at market restrictions, for example, we see how bird flu strategists began by promoting a value chain that would contain ducks within farm enclosures. The theory of containment, however, was soon abandoned when free-ranging ducks and farmers demonstrated their inextricability from the rice growing ecologies of the Mekong Delta. The endurance of unenclosed exchanges among ducks, rice, and farmers reflect the open-endedness and flexibility of experiments, and show how health subjects can change experimental conditions in situ.

Second, bird flu interventions take place in situations where biological objectives intersect with economic ones, which means that science is not the only system of knowledge and value shaping experiments. In Vietnamese livestock economies, public health agendas to control virus transmission intersect and collide with economic agendas that aim to increase poultry productivity. The NSCAI has chosen to promote an industrialized form of life in which poultry farming increases national GDP, and this means abandoning other forms of life that have sustained the livelihoods of the rural poor as well as the lives of non-commercial poultry. The economization of life that privileges market-oriented poultry producers *goes hand in hand* with a commoditization of life that privileges industrialized organisms. But the economization of life does not concern itself with income inequality, debt, or degrees of damage (Murphy 2017, 26–27), and as such farmers and fowl did not always comply with experimental interventions. Some farmers, like Trí and Thủy, chose to mix poultry breeds or dip halfway into commercial value chains while still maintaining their backyard farming systems. Others were like the model duck farmers in Đồng Tháp, who adopted new commercial life forms and exchange relations, but were hard pressed to continue with the experiment when their ducks failed to turn a profit. Despite NGO workers' efforts to couch the intervention in a discourse of health, not economics, farmers (and ducks) made their own responses to experimental conditions.

Third, bird flu experiments gather together a host of different actors and experts, who bring different ideas, practices, and ethical commitments to the table. Farmers and health professionals and vets and agricultural extension workers may disagree about what constitutes good health practice and good forms of poultry production and care. Where some might see free ranging behavior as imparting health and taste to animals, others may see the same experimental conditions as biological hazards. Poultry themselves may thwart intervention objectives, either by thrashing against vaccinators or failing to grow at industry standard rates. The behavior change campaign is one example of how different actors, knowledges, and practices collided in experimental interventions. While Cúc wanted to use participatory development frameworks to empower citizens to design their own behavioral changes, her collaborators insisted on social marketing principles that persuade health consumers to adopt predefined and quantifiable behaviors. Cúc was ultimately compelled to fall back on socialist state mobilization procedures and "trained" communities in healthy behaviors. The integration of different governing systems in this experiment was innovative, but it at the end of the day it circumscribed the extent to which vulnerable communities could shape their relationships with animals, environments, and authorities.

Taken together, bird flu interventions exemplify what Uli Biesel terms *real world experiments*: interventionist experiments that bleed into the broader social milieu in which they take place. Similar to the malaria control programs in Ghana that Biesel describes (2015), and the population control programs in Bangladesh that Michelle Murphy documents (2017), bird flu interventions see people and ideas transiting between arenas of scientific knowledge production, public health intervention, and sociocultural activity. Farms and markets, households and slaughterhouses, these sites are all subject to experimental exuberance. The dissolution of the boundary between experiment and world creates situations in which a whole host of actors, ideas, and organisms can influence the system. We saw how the mass vaccination campaign ended up enrolling more actors and ideas than initially intended. Paravets, family members, friends, neighbors, and fowl all weighed in on vaccination with their own theories about or experiences with infection, and their own techniques, practices, and technologies for managing it. In market interventions, farmers like Anh enrolled unsanctioned actors (family members) into commercial value chain labor, thereby altering the experiment in order to make it more do-able and family friendly. And in virus surveillance, virologists like Lee and Bảo bypassed global guidelines for sample sharing to generate more valuable data and benefits for Vietnam. These are experiments, then, with more than one active experimenter, and with inherently uncertain results (Biesel 2015, 293–95).

Understanding bird flu interventions as real world experimental systems is thus to situate them in larger assemblages of ideas, knowledge-practices, political-economic patterns, and cultural values (Rottenburg 2009). It is to attend to the broader social and cultural worlds that shape, and are shaped by, interventions. It is to recognize how experimental interventions rely on existing institutional and interpersonal relationships and exchanges to get things done.

Bird flu experiments may intervene in the real world, but their effects are not limited to the here and now. Like any experiment, HPAI interventions generate evidence for future experiments. It is important to ask how this evidence is collected and evaluated, especially in emergency situations where health programmers often act first and ask questions later. Vinh-Kim Nguyen argues that in situations of infectious disease crisis we see an inversion of the classical model of experiments, in which evidence of efficacy is generated under controlled conditions and then used to inform interventions. Nguyen uses the term "experimentality" to name experiments that move in the opposite direction. Experimentality, he says, intervenes first and then generates self-validating evidence ex post facto. This evidence, moreover, takes the form of "lessons learned," or "best practices" rather than any quantitative indication of health outcomes (2015, 71). In other words, the value of evidence lies in its ability to justify and perpetuate interventions, rather than to improve health.

The kind of evidentiary value Nguyen speaks of is visible in the Three Priority Behaviors Campaign. In this behavior change intervention, for-profit workers were preoccupied with generating evidence that showed how effective their messages were in reaching target audiences (not improving health outcomes). The evidence manifested in two ways: first in reports that counted the number of citizens exposed to the behavioral messages, and second in a pandemic simulation event where target audiences modeled the proposed behaviors for funders. Evidence here was valuable primarily to for-profit workers and their funders, for it demonstrated that project's marketing devices were an efficient use of donor funds. In what Alfred Montoya calls an "economy of virtue," the reports, images, and performances generated by the these types of multinational organizations acted as visible demonstrations of their virtue, and could be used to generate symbolic and real capital for future work (2012, 563). Importantly, these forms of evidence did not demonstrate any quantitative reductions in disease outbreaks, or even quantitative or qualitative indicators of whether or not individuals actually changed their behavior. It was of little direct value to anyone wanting to stem infection.

Similar forms of evidence making were apparent in the model duck biosecurity intervention, where NGO workers obtained data on farmers' compliance to biosecurity precepts in order to justify the costs of introducing the intervention elsewhere. Evidence here acted as a lubricant to ensure the continued flow of resources as experiments were scaled up and out. Importantly, these resources would not flow back to Đồng Tháp, instead evidentiary value flowed away from entrepreneurial farmers and ducks toward new experimental arenas. Evidence was valuable not in terms of improving health outcomes or poultry productivity in the here and now, but rather insofar as it showed that the experiments could travel (Petryna 2009).[1]

Because the value of experimental evidence was not always visible or beneficial to experimental subjects, value had to be found elsewhere. Bird flu programmers tried to frame value in terms of individual or household economic gain, rather than in terms of global health or the common good. Naturally Vietnam chicken producers, for instance, exchanged their animals for infection free local varieties and promises of increased profit and tastiness, thereby turning biosecurity risks into financial opportunities. Market reformers were enticed by small loans and stable work, and the prospect of being linked up with new commercial markets. These experimental subjects took a gamble on the idea that predefined commercial exchange relations would be better than independent and interpersonal ones, and that standardized, commercial poultry brands would be more profitable than native varieties. The value of these experiments lay in the fact that they facilitated new exchange relations; but in doing so they also put long-standing, socially significant exchange relations at risk. Anh, for instance, followed policies to commercialize his chicken holdings, but they strained his familial relations and compromised his family's rice production. Thủy and Trí followed national guidelines for the state provision of H5N1 vaccines, but they did so at the expense of the kin-based obligations that structured their practices of poultry care.

In response to the problematic outcomes of experimental exchanges, participants attempted to redirect value in experiments, and in ways that reflected culturally meaningful forms of giving and receiving in Vietnam. Farmers like Thủy and Trí drew on long-standing discourses of state patronage to make claims on vets for drug therapies. They and other farmers mobilized kin networks to address poultry illness and expand production, because they knew from experience the worth of affective exchanges among flocks and family. Hạnh and Thái requested NGO funds for model farmers in their district, thereby attempting to disrupt the flow of resources to scaled up interventions. Transnational scientists like Lee and Bảo expressed fidelity to existing forms of global virus exchange by sending samples to trusted agencies, even when they fell outside of recommended partnerships.

The ways in which participants maneuvered in bird flu interventions suggest that concepts often associated with global health experiments, like therapeutic domination and governmentality (Rottenburg 2009), fail to capture the diverse and enduring relations of obligation and care that animate multispecies life. The people I have described in this book often participated in interventions as risk-takers and entrepreneurs with a strong sense about what constitutes appropriate ways of living with disease risks and disease agents in Vietnam. And as experiments proceeded, they acted in accordance with empirical observations and historically and culturally inflected understandings about what works and what doesn't in livestock economies. In the everyday exchanges between humanitarian workers and for-profit consultants, paravets and poultry producers, virologists and farmers, family members and fowl, we can glimpse how different actors transformed experimental systems, generating and distributing value in locally significant ways.

Experimental value, then, can be deeply practical and empirical, but is also affective, bringing companion species, families, and community members together into relations of mutual dependence and care. Those involved in experimental interventions see risks, and promises, in the exchanges and connections they forge with different participants—whether human or nonhuman, local, state, or transnational. Although participants learned that there was no guarantee that they would benefit from an intervention, they sometimes found value in the experimetal encounter, creating wider connections with state and multinational institutions, health and development workers, commodity markets, and scientific centers. Frustrations and failure abounded, but participants also created new possibilities.

Experimental Futures

I want to end on this note of possibility. This book has been my attempt to upset the emerging standards and norms of One Health by presenting some alternatives. These alternatives are not my invention. Rather, I witnessed them surface on the ground, in the everyday process of health intervention, and in the everyday labor of poultry care. These alternatives—to model birds, to mass vaccination, to market restrictions, to moral instruction, and to material transfers—matter. They matter because they reveal *and reject* a key thread tying bird flu governance and its experimental multispecies exchange relations together: inequality. By inequality I mean the unequal distribution of resources to prevent flu infection in a pandemic age. I also mean the unequal valuation of life forms and forms of life in One Health programs that privilege certain futures over others.

Bird flu governance economizes life. It ties disease control to national and global economies by suggesting that health security can be found in poultry sector commercialization and industrialization. Within this view, the most efficient market actors are the safest; they are more valuable to the global economy and to global health. These are the lives worth safeguarding and propagating. Bird flu governance also ties disease control to particular forms of self-responsible health consumption, privileging those who are willing to bear more and more of the burden, and costs, of health care. As vaccines run dry and multinational assistance runs out, these entrepreneurial, self-regulating subjects are slated to be the ones engendering a flu-free future. In Vietnam, this means that the free-ranging, kin-based forms of life that have long characterized poultry production, and the socialized provisions that have long characterized state-society relations are being ignored, silenced, and trivialized under the norms of globalized bird flu control.

Undergirding the economization of life in bird flu governance is a commoditization of life that privileges some life forms over others. Though bird flu rhetoric celebrates local poultry, bird flu *interventions* privilege commercial varieties. Model ducks, model chickens, and market restrictions all constitute experiments to redefine which life forms can live to become commodities in Vietnamese poultry markets. These commoditization processes matter because they are impacting the future existence of entire poultry subspecies. They also matter because they limit the ability of many farmers to make do in a changing economy. Further, while novel global virus-sharing arrangements are changing the conditions under which human viruses become life saving commodities, animal viruses remain much less valuable and much less commoditizable. These variable virus commoditization processes matter because they reveal a devaluation of nonhuman animal life in a One Health arena that explicitly seeks to move beyond human exceptionalism. They also matter because undervaluing avian viruses limits the claims that nations like Vietnam will be able to make in market-driven global health orders.

Such are the norms and standards of One Health. But there are alternatives, and they can be found in the people, poultry, and pathogens described throughout this book: unflappable subjects, agents, and experts who searched for value and opportunities in inhospitable and relentlessly unequal conditions. I have tried to capture the dogged optimism and grit of state agents, the risk-taking entrepreneurialism of farmers, the fidelity of virus researchers, the compassion of NGO workers, and the agency of poultry and pathogens who, in spite of it all, continue to form meaningful and consequential biosocial attachments. By describing how different actors challenge the norms and reinvent the relations of bird flu governance, I have shown that One Health cannot and does not proceed from a fixed and universal biologic. Rather, One Health is constituted on the ground, in heterogeneous multispecies encounters and exchanges that bring biological concerns into generative conversation with economic, cultural, and moral ones. There is nothing singular about One Health.

In drawing attention to One Health's heterogeneity, this story makes room for new possibilities. The real world nature of bird flu experiments opens up opportunities for more actors to become experimenters weighing in on experimental design. There is an excess of risk-taking and ingenuity in Vietnam's livestock economies; it should be acknowledged and cultivated. I contend that One Health has to make room for agitation, questioning, innovation and alteration, not merely for the purposes of evidence collection, but as an actual form of engagement with and accountability to experimental communities—both human and nonhuman. I am calling for new forms of experimentation that celebrate, analyze, and even normalize the unanticipated responses of people, poultry and pathogens to experimental systems, rather than circumscribing them to the managerial language of lessons learned or cultural barriers. One Health must acknowledge and make room for alternative, *extra*-economic forms of value creation and multispecies exchange. It must open up avenues for a variety of participants to make demands upon experimental interventions. It must allow for the creation of new norms that are more in line with what matters to various actors in various locations. This may mean redistributing risk and opportunities in uncomfortable and uncontrollable ways. It may mean losing money, and maybe even lives.

The story of bird flu in Vietnam thus invites us to think about pandemics in terms of inequalities and not just threats. It invites us to look for, value, *and engage with* less visible and even less profitable life forms and forms of life in a pandemic age. I mean all of us: not just farmers, and not even just meat eaters, but anyone involved in any way in any food production system. Anyone who eats. Anyone who is vulnerable to a pandemic threat. Anyone who lives with others on this planet. The story of bird flu in Vietnam invites us to consider other ways of sustaining ourselves, of living together. Even if we don't adopt them, at the very least this story invites us to reject the *inevitability* of any "One" way of living with and killing others, and to be open to and permissive of alternatives. This is important, because the perceived inevitability of certain, "biosecure" life forms, certain forms of multispecies life, is a violent invention full of erasures and broken promises—with no guarantee for disease-free futures. Ultimately, the story of bird flu in Vietnam forces us to accept that we are all—human and nonhuman—implicated in the global regime of health experimentation. Let us therefore recuperate experiment, as a concept and a set of practices, through which we can imagine *and enact* more inclusive, more-than-human worlds.

Acknowledgments

I am grateful to the residents of Bắc Giang and Đồng Tháp provinces for their invaluable contributions to the research for this book. My biggest thanks goes to the Hoàng family in "Placid Pond" village, who took me in for several months and showed me nothing but patience, kindness, and generosity. Though their names have been changed in the text, these are people who taught me so very much, not least the meaning of *tình cảm*, moral sentiment. I am indebted to the Veterinary Administration of Đồng Tháp for offering logistical and administrative support for my research in the Mekong Delta. I am especially grateful to the provincial- and district-level veterinarians who worked tirelessly with me and abided my presence and participation in their already taxing work. In addition to supplying the empirical basis for much of this text, they offered friendship that saw me through long bouts of fieldwork. Representatives from Vietnam's Ministry of Health, Ministry of Agriculture and Rural Development, Department of Animal Health, Pasteur Institute, and National Institute of Health were generous with their time and resources. The Hanoi offices of the World Health Organization, Food and Agriculture Organization, UNICEF, and Abt Associates were also forthcoming with information and support, as were representatives from the World Health Organization in Geneva. For their hospitality and companionship during my stay in Vietnam, I would like to thank Nguyễn An Ninh, Dũng Tano, Lê Thị Thu, and Aphaluck Bhatiasevi.

The Department of Anthropology at the College of Social Sciences and Humanities, Vietnam National University–Hanoi, generously sponsored this research, and I am grateful to Professor Nguyễn Văn Sửu for his investment in and ongoing support of my scholarship. Lương Ngọc Vinh was instrumental in helping me navigate the landscape of research permissions and sponsorships in Vietnam.

Generous sources of funding over the years have made this book possible. Pilot research for this project was supported by a Robert Wood Johnson Health and Society Scholars Fellowship and a Scott Kloeck-Jensen International Pre-Dissertation Travel Grant. A Fulbright-Hays Doctoral Dissertation Research Award, a Social Science Research Council International Dissertation Grant, and a Wenner-Gren Foundation Dissertation Research Grant funded fieldwork in Vietnam. Data analysis and writing was funded by an Andrew W. Mellon/ACLS Dissertation Completion Fellowship and an Advanced Opportunity Fellowship from the University of Wisconsin–Madison. Further research support was provided by the European Research Council under the European Community's Seventh Framework Programme (FPT/2007–2019), ERC grant agreement no. 263447 (BioProperty). Support for the writing of this book was provided by the Wenner-Gren Foundation, with funding from the Hunt Postdoctoral Fellowship. A Brocher Foundation Visiting Research Fellowship also supported the writing of this book. The publication of this manuscript is made possible in part by support from the Institute for Scholarship in the Liberal Arts, College of Arts and Letters, University of Notre Dame.

I have presented material on this book in numerous presentations at the annual meetings of the American Anthropological Association and Society for the Social Studies of Sciences. I received generous suggestions for revising portions of the text from audiences at Durham University; Collège de France; the University of Hong Kong's Center for Humanities and Medicine; Goethe University; the University of Oslo's Institute for Technology, Innovation and Culture; University College London; Northwestern University; the University of Oxford; the University of Notre Dame; and the University of Wisconsin–Madison. Some of the arguments I make in this book are worked out in publications. Elements of chapter 2 appear in an article first published in *American Ethnologist* (Porter 2013), chapter 4 contains elements of an article published in *Sojourn: Journal of Social Issues in Southeast Asia* (Porter 2013), and portions of chapter 5 appear in an article published in *Public Culture* (Hinterberger and Porter 2015).

I have been privileged to work with wonderful mentors at the University of Wisconsin–Madison. Katherine Bowie taught me so many things, key among them the value of fieldwork. She offers the finest example of personally and politically invested, and accountable, anthropological research. She also taught me the delicate art of keeping crises at bay. Linda Hogle and Claire Wendland introduced me to science and technology studies and medical anthropology, and offered a model for mentorship that I strive to replicate.

Linda encouraged me to study avian flu and has been my most ardent sup-
porter. Claire strikes the perfect balance of critique and care, and has been
exceedingly generous with her time and counsel. I couldn't ask for better
teachers. Kenneth George, Paul Nadasdy, and Mark Sidel offered incisive
comments on the research, and Alfred McCoy and Ian Coxhead helped me
bring insights from history and economics to bear on the work.

I developed many of the ideas for this book as a research fellow of the
BioProperty Programme at the Institute of Science, Innovation and Society,
University of Oxford. As part of this fellowship, I engaged with an incredible
group of scholars who read and commented on early versions of this book,
and helped me develop my thinking toward issues of exchange, economy,
and property. Javier Lezaun, Amy Hinterberger, and Catherine Montgomery
were challenging and inspiring interlocutors. In our writing collaborations,
Amy and Javier pushed me to consider questions of sovereignty, animals,
containment, and ownership. It has been a privilege to write and think with
them. Steve Rayner, Idalina Baptista, Michele Acuto, Nils Markusson, Sophie
Haines, Ebru Soytemel, and Igor Calzada were delightful colleagues. My fellow writers at the Brocher Foundation gave thoughtful feedback on portions
of the text when I most needed it, and I am particularly grateful to Carl Hart,
Lingling Zhang, and Jane Davies for reminding me everyday of the value of
sincerity, and authenticity, in research and writing.

I would also like to thank Ilana Gershon, Kaushik Sunder Rajan, and
Allison Fish, who were kind enough to read and comment on the entire manuscript at various stages. Ilana's detailed attention to structure, style, and the big
picture greatly improved my writing and argumentation; and Kaushik's interventions encouraged me to clarify my intellectual framework and conceptual
contributions. I am grateful to both of them for their help with all aspects of
writing and publishing this book. Alex Nading, Fréderic Keck, and Ann Kelly
have shared insights with me on hosts, vectors, entanglements, and flu, and
I continue to learn from them and their work. I would also like to thank the
anonymous readers from the University of Chicago Press, whose feedback was
invaluable for developing the book's conceptual threads and situating them in
relation to different literatures. Lenore Manderson, Kimberly Guinta, and the
anonymous readers from Rutgers University were also instrumental to the
revision process. At the University of Chicago Press, I am indebted to Priya
Nelson, who patiently championed this project, and helped me unearth the
answers to its central questions. Thanks also to Dylan Montanari and Susan
Karani for their help with many of the details for publication.

I am grateful to my friends and colleagues for their ongoing engagement
with my work. Their questions, comments, and critiques have helped me see

this project through its long journey to publication. Thanks to Kristin Asdal, Sarah Besky, Nick Bingham, Alex Blanchette, Hannah Brown, Carlo Caduff, Haydon Cherry, Vivian Choi, Nicholas D'Avella, Thom van Doreen, Tone Druglitro, Anna Geltzer, Marion Girard-Dorsey, Sarah Grant, Kevin Hall, Jennifer Hamilton, Ellie Harrison-Buck, John Hartigan, Steve Hinchliffe, Meghan Howey, Ben Hurlbut, Frédéric Keck, Ann Kelly, Robert Kirk, Sabina Leonelli, Nadine Levin, Martha Lincoln, Celia Lowe, Christos Lynteris, Joe Lugalla, Linda Madsen, Michael Montesano, Christena Nippert-Eng, Juno Parrenas, Robert Peckham, Svetlana Peshkova, Julia Rodriguez, Susan Rottmann, Nick Shapiro, Robin Sheriff, Genese Sodikoff, Noah Tamarkin, Sara Withers, and Meike Wolf. My colleagues in the Anthropology Department at the University of Notre Dame have been essential to this project, and I would like to thank Susan Blum, Cat Bolten, Agustín Fuentes, Donna Glowacki, Lionel Jensen, Vania Smith-Oka, and Ann Marie Thornburgh, especially, for offering comments on parts of this book and giving sage advice on the publishing process. They are responsible for many of the insights found in this book, and none of its shortcomings.

Widely scattered friends have sustained me over the years. Thanks to Kyoko Arai, Chris Butler, Chisato Fukuda, Mark Golitko, Finn Golitko, Kari Heggelund, Khanthaly Koo, Hiro Nakano, Graham St. John, Katherine Thornton, Michiko Tsuneda, Emilie Utigard, Kirsten Warning, and Kent Wisniewski.

My family deserves my deepest gratitude. Robert Porter, Nathan Porter, Stacy Clinton, and the Haanstad, Walsh, and Pham families have always shown interest in and enthusiasm for this book, but thankfully never enough to provoke anxiety. Eric Haanstad saw this project from conception to completion, witnessed its lightest and darkest moments, and offered material and spiritual comfort, coffee and pancakes, just when I needed them. A special thanks to my canine companion, Nico, for always believing in me (I like to think). Finally, my parents, Dan and Hà Porter, have been with me all along, watching, waiting, reassuring, and encouraging. They embody *hy sinh*. This book is dedicated to them.

Notes

Introduction

1. In keeping with the nomenclature used by interlocutors at my research sites, throughout this book I use HPAI, H5N1, avian influenza, and bird flu to refer to highly pathogenic avian influenza.

2. Unless otherwise specified, the names of all people and villages in this account have been changed for privacy purposes. In Vietnamese, the modifier Ông precedes the names of respected men. It can signify man, husband, sir, or Mr. The modifier Bà precedes the name of respected women and signifies woman, wife, madam, or Mrs.

3. The regional differences in research conditions can be traced in part to the legacy of the Second Indochina War. The Communist administrative apparatus was developed and first implemented in the north, with cadres moving south to fill bureaucratic positions and instill Communist agendas in the "frontier" regions. As such, bureaucratic culture in the south tends to be much more restrictive and inflexible toward foreign researchers (Luong 2006). Research suggests that Communist cadres in the south tend to be more sedimented in policy and practice than those in the north, owing to their distance from the capital and their location in a more politically heterogeneous region (Taylor 2000).

4. Although large, commercialized operations have experienced the highest losses to HPAI in absolute terms, semi-commercial and backyard producers have suffered far greater losses relative to their income. Farmers for whom poultry is the primary source of income have suffered the most. In the small-scale sector, women, especially, lost poultry incomes and social standing, while backyard and semi-commercial producers suffered reduced access to urban markets (McLeod et al. 2006).

5. Under socialism, Vietnamese citizens received health care via a centralized, hierarchical public health system. Coverage was extensive and largely equitable, and free of charge. Although there were problems with efficiency and quality in the provision of health services, devices, and pharmaceuticals, under socialism Vietnamese citizens experienced relatively low mortality and morbidity rates in comparison with other so-called least developed nations (Fritzen 2007).

6. Susan Reynolds Whyte and her colleagues have shown a similar trend in Uganda. In what they term the "projectification" of AIDS care, they suggest that the Ugandan state has strategically utilized donor mobilization, or the establishment of myriad multinational projects for

HIV/AIDS prevention, eradication, and pharmaceutical development, as a means to retrench its national authority (Reynolds Whyte et al. 2013).

7. Though it has roots in nineteenth-century comparative medicine, One Health today proceeds from concerns about emerging and reemerging infectious diseases that have multiple hosts and multiple vectors. These diseases include HPAI, SARS, Ebola, monkey pox, and West Nile fever.

8. To address bird flu, for instance, the World Health Organization, the World Organization for Animal Health, and the Food and Agricultural Organization signed an agreement to share responsibilities for managing health activities at the human-animal-ecosystems interface (Food and Agriculture Organization, World Health Organization, and World Organization for Animal Health 2010).

9. Global designs toward biosecurity work in tandem with a Vietnamese governmental strategy to prepare domestic poultry production for eventual adoption in global livestock markets—this despite evidence that commercial, industrial production systems engender higher risks for H5N1 and other communicable diseases (Davis 2005).

10. For instance, Nicole Shukin (2009) has shown how modern societies are built on *animal capital*. The materials from animals and animal labor create wealth, while animals themselves obtain a variety of cultural meanings—many of which are associated with the exploitation of certain groups of people.

11. Scholars in anthropology and science and technology studies have explored experiments and experimentation in a number of domains, from clinical trials to medical research and public health practice (Sunder Rajan 2006, 2017; Geissler 2015; Geissler and Kelly 2016; Petryna 2009; Nelson 2013; Nguyen 2009, 2015; Porter 2015; Rottenburg 2009; Murphy 2017; Kohler 1994; Creager 2001; Davies 2012, 2013).

12. There is a rich anthropological body of research on the advances and missteps of multispecies health interventions for zoonotic and vector-borne diseases (Nading 2014a; Kelly and Lezaun 2013; Lezaun and Porter 2015; Brown and Kelly 2014; Zhan 2005; Biesel 2015; Fearnley 2015, 2018; Keck 2008, 2014, 2015).

Gà Ta, Our Chicken

1. Charles Darwin was an early proponent of the theory that the domestic chicken originated from the Southeast Asian Red Jungle Fowl. This theory has recently been complicated by accounts suggesting that the modern chicken originates from several varieties of jungle fowl found in Asia, which may have also crossbred with varieties from Europe or the Americas (Smith and Daniel 2000, 27–30).

2. Prior to French colonization, local leaders established military-agricultural settlements in uncultivated areas and recruited peasants to work on plantations by granting titles to the lands they cleared (Ho Tai and Sidel 2012, 3–9).

Chapter One

1. For a discussion on ethnographic approaches to nonhuman forms of life, see Hartigan 2015.

2. The same principle is also applied to humans. When I fell ill in Placid Pond, Thủy sent her daughter, Qui, out to buy acetaminophen because she feared my body would not respond

to Chinese medicine *(thuốc bắc)*. Such associations between bodies and geography play a part in farmers' risk-taking decisions about whether and how to raise new, biosecure poultry breeds.

3. The Vietnamese farm has long served as a site for health engineering and the management of intersections between human and nonhuman organisms in rural space. To give one example, malaria control expertise in colonial Vietnam centered on models of biophysical environments in which plasmodia moved from mosquitoes to humans and back again. Operating on the assumption that, like bird flu viruses, malaria constantly circulates in farming ecologies, disease strategists proposed targeted, bodily measures to prevent infection at the species interface, including mosquito nets, quinine, and insect population reduction. What's more, these disease control strategies were couched in rhetoric of peasant self-development and "human capital." Such development-oriented health agendas that continued to gain force in the postcolonial era as revolutionary medicine encouraged villagers to abandon their "superstitions" and regulate their interactions with infectious agents through hygiene practices and mosquito elimination (Malarney 2007; Aso 2013). Narrated as part of a larger effort to improve the conditions of the peasantry, infectious disease control in rural Vietnam links environmental and social engineering processes to ideas of human development and farmer empowerment.

4. By "regime of value," I refer to theoretical discussions about the shifting value of commodities as they move across different spaces and exchange relations. Arjun Appadurai uses the concept to encourage anthropologists to trace commodities as they pass through site-specific systems of meaning, and to look for the value ascribed to them in this process (1988, 5). Kaushik Sunder Rajan develops this concept in his work on biomedical research and the pharmaceutical industry, showing how biomaterials, data, and drug therapies gain economic, moral, and scientific value in different geopolitical locations, which have their own locally specific institutional and juridical cultures and practices—even as they are linked up to global research and market networks (2006, 2017).

Hatching

1. Drawing on Evans-Pritchard's account and her own ethnographic research, Sharon Hutchinson notes a similar process among the Nuer of Southern Sudan, where "a fundamental 'oneness' between cattle and people . . . enabled people to extend the potency of human action in tempering the perplexing vicissitudes and vulnerabilities of life" (Hutchinson 1992, 296).

Chapter Two

1. The first line defense against infectious livestock diseases, stamping out (or culling flocks displaying symptoms of infection) did not eliminate the H5N1 HPAI virus. This failure can be traced in part to the fact that reporting and surveillance systems in Vietnam do not capture all cases of infection. There are several reasons for this: (1) not all small farmers report disease; (2) relationships among veterinary officials and poultry farmers are often weak; (3) some infected poultry (particularly ducks) do not display clinical signs of infection; (4) infected poultry in live bird markets may go unnoticed; (5) inadequate field and laboratory capacity impede surveillance and disease tracing; (6) the pressures to control known outbreaks hinder disease investigations and epidemiological tracing; (7) Vietnam's complex poultry market chains make tracing infections difficult (Sims and Do 2009; Ministry of Health and Ministry of Agriculture and Rural Development 2010).

2. This despite the fact that in 2010, Vietnam's H5N1 viral strain began showing signs of mutating into a more lethal form immune to the vaccine being used in the country (H5N1 Re-5) (Phan 2011). The OIE characterized the new virus as H5N1 clade 2.3.2.1 (World Organization for Animal Health 2011).

3. Notably, these ideas about the misappropriation of vaccines contrast with external assessments of Vietnam's veterinary sector. A comprehensive assessment of Vietnam's veterinary services prepared by the OIE reported relatively good compliance of registration and use of vet pharmaceutical products, including vaccines (Fermet-Quinet, Jane, and Forman 2007).

4. In Vietnam, private veterinarians do not have access to delegation of public duties, but, according to OIE estimates, two-thirds of them have contractual links with public services (Fermet-Quinet, Edan, and Stratton 2010).

5. For a discussion of the organizing force of this adage in the practice of medicine in Vietnam, see Craig 2002, p. 190.

6. Experts have been cautious in their response to these figures. For example, Sims and Do (2009) note that it is not known whether these reductions were a direct result of vaccination, a coincidence, or the consequence of other control measures. Most assessments agree that the drops in infection rates after vaccination have occurred as a result of using vaccination in conjunction with other measures including disinfection, movement control, and market regulations (Ministry of Health and Ministry of Agriculture and Rural Development 2010).

Chapter Three

1. In this case 99 Poultry, a Vietnamese conglomerate headquartered in the Biên Hòa industrial zone approximately forty kilometers east of Ho Chi Minh City.

2. Eight markets serving the three provinces of Hà Tây, Hà Nam, and Hanoi absorb birds from a total population of almost four hundred Sector 3 farms (260000 birds/year) (Otte et al. 2008, 9). The money that agricultural producing families make from selling flocks in city markets represents a large proportion of their total assets (Mcleod, Thieme, and Mack 2009, 192). As agricultural space in and around Hanoi and Ho Chi Minh City is being restructured and reallotted for industrial and financial endeavors, urban consumers primarily purchase from producers outside of the city.

3. Even before bird flu viruses appeared in Hanoi, Vietnamese scholars and leaders had been warning that cities were under threat of ruralization (*nông thôn hoá*), or the incursion of rural activities and actors into urban areas space. They had also expressed concerns about rural health problems emerging from the infiltration of new pests in agricultural space and alterations in air quality brought about by urban expansion (Harms 2011, 18). The environmental concerns raised by ongoing ecological transformations include not only the displacement of peri-urban agricultural zones, but also the possibility of more weakly enforced environmental regulations as industrial activities become dispersed across a wider territory, and in many cases hidden by myriad other land uses at the urban edge (Leaf 1999).

4. This market restriction policy has been carried out differently in Hanoi and Ho Chi Minh City. In 2005, both Hanoi and Ho Chi Minh City authorities banned poultry production, live markets, and processing in urban areas during bird flu outbreaks. Yet only authorities in Ho Chi Minh City continued to enforce the ban after the early outbreak periods (2004–5) ended. In contrast, Hanoi city authorities relaxed quarantine measures taken during outbreaks and permitted the marketing chain to revert to pre-outbreak systems early on (Otte 2007).

5. According to Agrifood Consulting International, Hà Vĩ market averaged around 300 tons

of chicken and 100 tons of duck per month prior to avian flu outbreaks in 2005. In July 2006 Hà Vĩ's volume of monthly trade shrunk to 150 tons and 80 tons per month, respectively. The main suppliers were the Thai and Japanese conglomerates, CP and JAPFA, as well as larger commercial and semi-commercial farms in Hà Tây, Hưng Yên and Hải Dương provinces. CP and JAPFA had around 30 percent of the market, while forty large assemblers and wholesalers had another 40 percent and the remaining share of the market comprised around forty smaller assemblers and wholesalers. Further, sales of poultry from Hà Vĩ market are to mainly Hanoi (70 percent), with the remainder of being sold within Hà Tây Province, predominantly to Hà Đông township. The volume of trade with Hanoi has reduced substantially, particularly during the HPAI outbreaks when trade was restricted. Post HPAI, trade requires veterinary clearances from the commune level (10,000 dong per truck—about 80 cents) and from the provincial department (20,000 dong per truck) (Agrifood Consulting International 2007, 210–11).

6. The risks of industrial ecosystems are twofold: first, high concentrations of poultry infected by wild avian viruses become passage points through which HPAI transmits to human poultry workers; second, high-density poultry flocks also act as loci of pathogen evolution, as wild-type avian viruses adapt to humans during replication in poultry (Leibler et al. 2009, 2). What's more, outside of direct people to poultry contact, industrial-integrated ecosystems provide a number of unrecognized and unregulated pathways for pathogen transfer, including airborne dust, nuisance insects, animal wastes, contaminated water, and interloping wild animals.

7. The productive contrast between rural (*nông thôn*) and urban (*thành thị*) aligns with what some scholars have called the dual cosmos in Vietnamese structures of thinking, where the opposing forces of *âm | dương* (yin | yang) organize aspects of everyday life such as economic activities, public conduct, and interpersonal relations (Jamieson 1995). These theories of Vietnamese thought and action are largely discounted today.

8. In addition to providing fiscal incentives for small-scale and household poultry producers to replace their flocks with other livestock or agricultural goods, in some provinces the Vietnamese government has offered loans for farmers to relocate to agricultural zones where they could engage in mixed farming. Denoted VAT (vườn áp, trai—garden, pond, farm), such mixed farms combined fruit, fish, and livestock in an attempt to reduce the density of poultry in villages, and to dilute the risks farmers would face in the event of a disease outbreak or market shock for any one product.

9. These production patterns resonate with what Lyle Fearnley (2018), expanding on Li Huaiyin's analysis, describes for duck farming in bird flu affected southern China. He characterizes duck farming as an incorporation of sideline (noncommercial, supplementary) and business farming (generating most of the family income) following farm decollectivization, rather than a transition from one to the other.

10. To Xuan Phuc (2011) provides an illuminating account of the rural-urban penetrations flowing in the opposite direction, showing that as rich urban dwellers vacation in the countryside, they build holiday homes and infrastructures that transform landscapes and social dynamics.

Chapter Four

1. These refrains come from UNICEF's Avian and Pandemic Influenza Communications Resources Division. They appear in a leaflet entitled, "Bài Em Học Hôm Nay: Vệ Chăn Nuôi Gia Cầm," or "Pocket Poultry Raising Guide." In an effort to maintain the rhyming verse from the Vietnamese, the English versions of these pamphlets contain interpretive translations of

Vietnamese text. Here I include more literal translations that differ somewhat from the more poetic, published English versions. Notably, in the first message, the English translation adds the statement, "Be a good farmer," which does not appear in the Vietnamese version. I include the statement here in order to signal that farmers are the target audience for the messages.

2. The bureau was established by the DRV President Ho Chi Minh's national liberation front, the Việt Minh (the League of Independence of Vietnam).

3. Many artists from the Hanoi College of Fine Arts volunteered to go south to support the war effort against the French and then later against the Americans. Artists lived on the frontlines with soldiers, set up art classes at the jungle headquarters of the National Liberation Front of South Vietnam, and fought and died in battle. As one artist noted, "In those days you contributed your whole life to the revolution without ever asking for recognition" (quoted in Taylor 2004, 29).

4. Professors from the Soviet Union taught at the College of Fine Arts in Hanoi, and students were regularly sent to Soviet universities in Moscow, Leningrad, and Kiev to learn the principles and techniques of the genre. As the artists completed their training, socialist realist propaganda became more prominent. When the DRV set its sights on reunifying the country after the First Indochina War, more and more artists found employment—as illustrators for the state-controlled press, and as poster designers for the government's "advertising" campaigns (see Taylor 2004).

5. Such artistic representations were effective. An estimated one million women fought on the frontline and supported the war effort. Karen Turner (1999) suggests that in doing so, revolutionary fighters not only followed nationalistic directives, but also drew on a historical pantheon in which heroic women mounted elephants and engaged in spectacular battles against Chinese invaders in order to defend their husbands and nation. This tradition is encapsulated by a well-known Vietnamese adage that states, "When war strikes close to home, even the women must fight."

6. Vietnam has a long history of female involvement in revolutionary struggle. The most famous of which are the legendary Trưng sisters. Vietnamese historians assert that the Chinese killed Trưng Trác's husband, the Vietnamese lord Thị Sách. In avenging his death, she and her sister violently rebelled against and defeated the Chinese, establishing their own kingdom over which they reigned as queens. Patricia Pelley writes, "In resisting the Han Chinese, they rehearsed what later became the essential drama: the expulsion of aggressive foreigners from the sacred land of Vietnam. As that model was periodically restaged, successive heroes and successive struggles reenacted the 'immortal spirit,' that had passed, beginning with the Trung sisters in 40 C.E., from one generation of Vietnamese to the next. In the twentieth century, thanks to the 'bright light' of 'Uncle Ho,' the Communist Party, and the People's arm, the Vietnamese would bring to fruition what the two sisters had begun" (Pelley 2002, 181).

7. In a similar analysis of modernizing public health agendas in revolutionary China, Ruth Rogaski (2004) develops the concept of hygienic modernity to illustrate the deployment of state agendas to develop national strength through population-centered health campaigns such as vaccinations.

8. People's Committee offices are local organs of state administration, and they incorporate a variety of staff, including veterinary and public health agents who carry out government policies within their jurisdictions. Mass organizations are technically nongovernmental and were developed by the Communist Party as an apparatus to implement government policy at the local level. In organizations like the Vietnam Farmer's Union, the Vietnam Women's Union, and

the Vietnam Youth Union, volunteer brigades visit households to introduce governmental edicts relevant to their various demographics (Salemink 2006). People's Committees offices and mass organizations are both organized from the central government down to the provincial, district, commune, and hamlet levels, and they receive the majority if not all of their funding from the state budget (Fforde 2005).

9. Summerson Carr (2009) refers to these processes as anticipatory interpellation. Individuals anticipate how interveners view them, and what interveners want from them, and respond from their designated positions as empowered, yet uneducated community members in order to make socioeconomic requests.

10. In combining ethnographic and genealogical approaches, I take inspiration from Ann Marie Leshkowich's (2014) study of standardized forms and documents in Vietnam.

Chapter Five

1. The WHO narrates the origins of global influenza virus surveillance as far back as the 1918 pandemic flu (Spanish Flu). According to this narrative, the devastation caused by this infection prompted the US and the UK to begin informally collecting seasonal flu virus samples from countries around the world so that they could be characterized and monitored for potentially dangerous mutations, and so that the most effective seasonal vaccines could be developed. Notably, the early period of virus surveillance saw most of the samples moving between countries in the Global North where influenza was thought to be more prevalent.

2. While the CBD affords nations the right to determine the terms of access to "their" biological resources, it prohibits them from being "unreasonably" restrictive (Hayden 2003, 64). Sovereignty here does not signal exclusive ownership but rather acts as a tool to manage resource exchange.

3. This notion of viruses as a common global threat was codified in the revised International Health Regulations for WHO member states, which posits the obligations of nation-states to accept global intervention in a context of the heightened pathogen circulation.

4. PIP includes an SMTA that prohibits those providing or receiving the virus within the network to seek any intellectual property on *human* clinical specimens, virus isolates of pandemic potential, and modified viruses prepared from influenza virus sample (World Health Organization 2011, Article 6.1). A second SMTA establishes a mechanism for granting nonexclusive licenses to at-risk, resource poor countries for the production of patented vaccines and other products in the event of a pandemic. It also requests that pharmaceutical industry manufacturers donate a percentage of their vaccines and antiviral treatments to the WHO for distribution to at-risk nations, and that they provide vaccines and antiviral treatments at affordable prices to them (World Health Organization 2011, Article 4.A6). The PIP framework further calls for the inclusion of scientists from developing countries in research and publication on the viruses (World Health Organization 2011, Articles 6 and 2).

5. In making a distinction between the informational and material status of viruses, I do not mean to imply that data lacks materiality. Much work has been done in science and technology studies to demonstrate data's material aspects and material cultures surrounding Big Data (Lupton 2016; Pink et al. 2018; Pink, Ardèvol, and Lanzeni 2016; Leonardi 2010; Tanweer, Fiore-Gartland, and Aragon 2016). I also do not mean to suggest that virus sequence data travels more easily or freely than samples. Data dissemination on a global scale requires a politics of coordination (Hilgartner 2013), in which well-coordinated networks of individuals, scientific

communities, companies, and institutions take responsibility for developing, financing, and regulating data infrastructures (Leonelli 2016).

6. The imperative to share in biomedicine coincides with a perceived "market failure" for pharmaceuticals and the establishment of new resource-sharing arrangements among the pharmaceutical industry, academia, government, and philanthropic organizations. These arrangements that seek to address the limitations of state, non-state, and corporate actors working independently. Sharing is also situated in a global health order, which posits that health issues transcend national territories and cannot fall under the purview of states alone. However, rather than ensure equal access to resources or build state capacity, a kind of "scientific sovereignty" has emerged in global health and biomedical "collaborations," wherein private entities and non-governmental and supranational organizations compete with states in the provision of health services (Samsky 2012). At the same time, individuals are asserting citizenship claims in relation to transnational rather than state actors, claims that rest on biological (Petryna 2002; Novas and Rose 2005) and therapeutic (Nguyen 2005) conditions rather than national identities. It is in the context of these trends that viral ownership claims disrupts the imperative to share, by pointing out that sharing does not necessarily benefit more vulnerable partners in health collaborations.

7. Though publicly available, online repositories of sequence information are not accessible to all, and many countries in the Global South do not have the technical capabilities to access these databases (Leonelli 2016).

8. It is curious that, even though Indonesia stopped forwarding poultry viruses to OFFLU around the same time that it ceased sharing human samples with the WHO, Siti Fadilah Supari did not call for new benefit-sharing agreements from the OIE/FAO. Analysts suggest that the reason for this disconnect in animal virus sharing was due to the fact that Indonesia was ignoring the animal health side of pandemic preparedness. WATTAGNet, a consortium on global poultry animal feed industries, reported, "Indonesia appears to have given up on surveillance, identification and documentation of H5N1 outbreaks in poultry, as seen by inability to link one third of recent human cases to poultry. Indonesian reports on other cases simply contain some vague reference to sick or dying fowls in the affected area" (Mabbett 2009, "H5N1 Sample Hoarding").

9. Baxter, Sanofi-Pasteur, Pfizer, and other major pharmaceutical corporations have raced to develop human pandemic flu vaccines, and competition over scarce supplies has made national stockpiles a matter of state secrecy. Conversely, the companies manufacturing poultry vaccines are much more diversified, with scores of laboratories across affected nations obtaining licenses for production.

10. For instance, in the spring of 2015, a major bird flu outbreak devastated poultry flocks in the Midwestern United States and prompted the destruction of over thirteen million birds. While poultry producers requested the production of an H5N2 vaccine to stem infections, regulators from the CDC called these interventions unrealistic. One official stated, "So far, there is no reason to believe that H5 could not be controlled through culling," and sanitary precautions aimed at keeping environmental viruses out of henhouses (MacKenzie 2015).

11. There are signs, however, that the role of poultry vaccination may be changing in global health efforts against avian flu. In May 2015, researchers from Kansas State University and the US Department of Homeland Security developed vaccines for H5N1 and H7N9 using strains from Egypt, Indonesia, and other Southeast Asian and North African countries. The researchers used recombinant technology to transplant sections of H5N1 and H7N9 into a Newcastle virus vaccine. The resulting vaccine was protective against all three diseases (Liu et al. 2015).

Conclusion

1. As experiments travel to different sites, the kinds of evidentiary value they generate can take unexpected form. Adriana Petryna has argued that experimental drug trials display ethical variability. Particularly in situations of state withdrawal, compromised health infrastructures, and patchy ethical oversight, experimentality creates its own measures of success by taking the difficult realities of local contexts and capacities as a basis upon which to "work ethics" (Petryna 2009, 30). What she means by this is that experimental designers might take recalcitrant, difficult, or otherwise unexpected experimental conditions in resource-poor areas as justification for altering global ethical principles for medical research. If, for example, the material or human resources at experimental sites are unavailable, or if legal frameworks for protecting human subjects do not exist at the national level, then ethical guidelines can be fudged in order to cater to "local conditions." This, of course, is a dangerous game, and often results in negative and sometimes disastrous health consequences for experimental subjects. In Vietnam, ethical variability allows designers of experimental interventions to extract value from them, even when they have ambiguous local effects. For instance, the patchy distribution of flu vaccines has become part of a longer-term governmental effort for building veterinarian's capacity to reach citizens; farmers' aversion to commercial poultry production has prompted multinational advisors to call for alternative conduits to commercialization, such as Naturally Vietnam chickens; for-profit firm representatives interpreted focus groups' lukewarm response to behavior change messaging as a first step in persuading them to take responsibility for health; and NGO representatives celebrated model farms not for improving incomes but rather for creating a baseline study for repeating the intervention elsewhere. The ways in which flu strategists worked ethics might have been innovative and adaptive, but they still clung to predetermined objectives and indicators of value that failed to attend to the needs and conditions of experimental subjects.

References

Adams, Vincanne, Thomas Novotny, and Hannah Leslie. 2008. "Global Health Diplomacy." *Medical Anthropology* 27 (4): 315–23.

Agrifood Consulting International. 2006. *The Impact of Avian Influenza on Poultry Sector Restructuring and Its Socio-Economic Effects.* Report prepared for the Food and Agriculture Organization of the United Nations by Agrifood Consulting International, USA. http://www.fao.org/docs/eims/upload//211945/Impact_of_AI_on_Poultry_Market_Chains-final_report.pdf. Accessed May 11, 2012.

———. 2007. "The Economic Impact of Highly Pathogenic Avian Influenza: Related Biosecurity Policies on the Vietnamese Poultry Sector." Report prepared for the Food and Agriculture Organization of the United Nations and the World Health Organization by Agrifood Consulting International, USA.

Allen, John, and Stephanie Lavau. 2015. "'Just-in-Time' Disease." *Journal of Cultural Economy* 8 (3): 342–60. https://doi.org/10.1080/17530350.2014.904243.

Anderson, Warwick. 2006. *Colonial Pathologies: American Tropical Medicine, Race, and Hygiene in the Philippines.* Durham, NC: Duke University Press.

Ankeny, Rachel A., Sabina Leonelli, Nicole C. Nelson, and Edmund Ramsden. 2014. "Making Organisms Model Human Behavior: Situated Models in North-American Alcohol Research, since 1950." *Science in Context* 27 (3): 485–509.

Appadurai, Arjun, ed. 1988. *The Social Life of Things: Commodities in Cultural Perspective.* Cambridge: Cambridge University Press.

Aso, Michitake. 2013. "Patriotic Hygiene: Tracing New Places of Knowledge Production about Malaria in Vietnam, 1919–75." *Journal of Southeast Asian Studies* 44: 423–43. Singapore: Cambridge University Press.

Baynes-Rock, Marcus. 2015. *Among the Bone Eaters: Encounters with Hyenas in Harar.* University Park, PA: Penn State University Press.

Bellacasa, María Puig de la. 2012. "'Nothing Comes without Its World': Thinking with Care." *Sociological Review* 60 (2): 197–216. https://doi.org/10.1111/j.1467-954X.2012.02070.x.

Benezra, Amber. 2016. "Datafying Microbes: Malnutrition at the Intersection of Genomics and Global Health." *BioSocieties* 11 (3): 334–51. https://doi.org/10.1057/biosoc.2016.16.

———. 2017. "Writing the Microbiome: Medical Anthropology Quarterly." *Medical Anthro-*

pology Quarterly (blog). June 10. http://medanthroquarterly.org/2017/06/10/writing-the
-microbiome/. Accessed June 2, 2018.

Biehl, Joao. 2006. "Pharmaceutical Governance." In *Global Pharmaceuticals: Ethics, Markets, Practices,* edited by Andrew Lakoff, Adriana Petryna, and Arthur Kleinman, 206–40. Durham, NC: Duke University Press.

Biesel, Ulrike. 2015. "The Blue Warriors: Ecology, Participation, and Public Health in Malaria Control Experiments." In *Para-States and Medical Science: Making African Global Health,* edited by Paul Wenzel Geissler, 281–302. Durham, NC: Duke University Press.

Biesel, Ulrike, and Christophe Boete. 2013. "The Flying Public Health Tool: Genetically Modified Mosquitoes and Malaria Control." *Science as Culture* 22 (1): 38–60.

Biggs, David. 2003. "Problematic Progress: Reading Environmental and Social Change in the Mekong Delta." *Journal of Southeast Asian Studies* 34 (1): 77–96.

Blanchette, Alex. 2015. "Herding Species: Biosecurity, Posthuman Labor, and the American Industrial Pig." *Cultural Anthropology* 30 (4): 640–69. https://doi.org/10.14506/ca30.4.09.

———. 2018. "How to Act Industrial around Industrial Pigs." In *Living with Animals: Bonds across Species,* edited by Natalie Porter and Ilana Gershon. Ithaca, NY: Cornell University Press.

Branswell, Helen. 2007. "Poor Countries Insisting on Bird Flu Rules: They Want Fair Share of Vaccines." *Hamilton Spectator,* February 12, sec. A.

Braun, Bruce. 2007. "Biopolitics and the Molecularization of Life." *Cultural Geographies* 14 (1): 6–28. https://doi.org/10.1177/1474474007072817.

Briggs, Charles L., and Mark Nichter. 2009. "Biocommunicability and the Biopolitics of Pandemic Threats." *Medical Anthropology* 28 (3): 189–98. https://doi.org/10.1080/0145974090 3070410.

Brown, Hannah, and Ann H. Kelly. 2014. "Material Proximities and Hotspots: Toward an Anthropology of Viral Hemorrhagic Fevers." *Medical Anthropology Quarterly* (April). https:// doi.org/10.1111/maq.12092.

Buchanan, David R., Sasiragha Reddy, and Zafar Hossain. 1994. "Social Marketing: A Critical Appraisal." *Health Promotion International* 9 (1): 49–57. https://doi.org/10.1093/heapro/ 9.1.49.

Buller, Henry. 2013. "Individuation, the Mass and Farm Animals." *Theory, Culture & Society* 30 (7–8): 155–75. https://doi.org/10.1177/0263276413501205.

Bulmer, R. 1973. "Why the Cassowary Is Not a Bird." In *Rules and Meanings: The Anthropology of Everyday Knowledge; Selected Readings,* edited by Mary Douglas. Harmondsworth, UK: Penguin.

Buse, Kent, and Gill Walt. 1997. "An Unruly Melange? Coordinating External Resources to the Health Sector: A Review." *Social Science & Medicine* 45 (3): 449–63.

———. 2002. "The World Health Organization and Global Public-Private Partnerships: In Search of 'Good' Global Governance." In *Public-Private Partnerships for Public Health,* edited by Michael Reich, 169–95. Cambridge, MA: Harvard University Press.

Cadena, Marisol de la. 2015. *Earth Beings: Ecologies of Practice across Andean Worlds.* Durham, NC: Duke University Press.

Caduff, Carlo. 2012. "The Semiotics of Security: Infectious Disease Research and the Biopolitics of Informational Bodies in the United States." *Cultural Anthropology* 27 (2): 333–57. https:// doi.org/10.1111/j.1548-1360.2012.01146.x.

———. 2014. "Pandemic Prophecy, or How to Have Faith in Reason." *Current Anthropology* 55 (3): 296–315. https://doi.org/10.1086/676124.

————. 2015. *The Pandemic Perhaps: Dramatic Events in a Public Culture of Danger*. Oakland: University of California Press.

CARE International Vietnam. 2006. "Avian Influenza Local Risk Reduction Project Baseline KAP Study." Unpublished research report. Hanoi: Vietnam.

Carr, Summerson. 2009. "Anticipating and Inhabiting Institutional Identities." *American Ethnologist* 36 (2): 317–36. https://doi.org/10.1111/j.1548-1425.2009.01137.x.

Chaudhuri, Anoshua, and Kakoli Roy. 2008. "Changes in Out-of-Pocket Payments for Healthcare in Vietnam and Its Impact on Equity in Payments, 1992–2002." *Health Policy (Amsterdam, Netherlands)* 88 (1): 38–48. https://doi.org/10.1016/j.healthpol.2008.02.014.

Chen, Lincoln, and Linda Hiebert. 1994. "From Socialism to Private Markets: Vietnam's Health in Rapid Transition." http://www.hawaii.edu/hivandaids/From_Socialism_To_Private_Markets_Vietnam_s_Health_In_Rapid_Transition.pdf. Accessed July 8, 2010.

Chiew, Florence. 2014. "Posthuman Ethics with Cary Wolfe and Karen Barad: Animal Compassion as Trans-Species Entanglement." *Theory, Culture & Society* 31 (4): 51–69. https://doi.org/10.1177/0263276413508449.

Choy, Timothy K. 2005. "Articulated Knowledges: Environmental Forms after Universality's Demise." *American Anthropologist* 107 (1): 5–18.

Cohen, Ed. 2011. "The Paradoxical Politics of Viral Containment; or, How Scale Undoes Us One and All." *Social Text* 29 (1) (106): 15–35. https://doi.org/10.1215/01642472-1210247.

Comaroff, John L., and Jean Comaroff. 1990. "Goodly Beasts, Beastly Goods: Cattle and Commodities in a South African Context." *American Ethnologist* 17: 195–216.

Cook, Robert A., William B. Karesh, and Steven A. Osofsky. 2009. "One World, One Health." Organization. One World, One Health. 2009. http://www.oneworldonehealth.org. Accessed September 6, 2013.

Craig, David. 2002. *Familiar Medicine: Everyday Health Knowledge and Practice in Today's Vietnam*. Honolulu: University of Hawai'i Press.

Craig, David, and Doug Porter. 2006. "Vietnam: Framing the Community, Clasping the People." In *Development beyond Neoliberalism? Governance, Poverty Reduction and Political Economy*, edited by David Craig and Doug Porter, 125–54. New York: Routledge.

Creager, Angela. 2001. *The Life of a Virus*. Chicago: University of Chicago Press.

Csordas, Thomas. 2011. "Cultural Phenomenology: Embodiment, Agency, Sexual Difference, and Illness." In *A Companion to the Anthropology of the Body and Embodiment*, edited by Frances E. Mascia-Lees, 137–56. Hoboken, NY: Wiley.

Dang, Nguyen Anh. 1999. "Market Reforms and Internal Labor Migration in Vietnam." *Asian and Pacific Migration Journal* 8 (3): 381–407.

Das, Veena. 1998. "Wittgenstein and Anthropology." *Annual Review of Anthropology* 27: 171–95.

————. 2016. "The Boundaries of the 'We': Cruelty, Responsibility and Forms of Life." *Critical Horizons* 17 (2): 168–85. https://doi.org/10.1080/14409917.2016.1153888.

Davies, Gail. 2011. "Writing Biology with Mutant Mice: The Monstrous Potential of Post Genomic Life." *Geoforum* (April). https://doi.org/10.1016/j.geoforum.2011.03.004.

————. 2012. "What Is a Humanized Mouse? Remaking the Species and Spaces of Translational Medicine." *Body & Society* 18 (3–4): 126–55. https://doi.org/10.1177/1357034X12446378.

————. 2013. "Writing Biology with Mutant Mice: The Monstrous Potential of Post Genomic Life." *Geoforum* 48 (August): 268–78. https://doi.org/10.1016/j.geoforum.2011.03.004.

Davis, Mike. 2005. *The Monster at Our Door: The Global Threat of Avian Flu*. New York: New Press.

Defossez, Ellen. 2016. "Health and Personal Responsibility in the Context of Neoliberalism:

Cultivating Alertness, Autonomy and Accountability through Three Contemporary Health Practices," no. 9: 7.

Delgado, C. L., M. W. Rosegrant, and S. Meijer. 2002. "Livestock to 2020: The Revolution Continues." International Trade in Livestock Products Symposium, January 18–19, 2002, Auckland, New Zealand 14560. International Agricultural Trade Research Consortium.

Despret, Vinciane. 2004. "The Body We Care For: Figures of Anthropo-Zoo-Genesis." *Body & Society* 10 (2–3): 111–34. https://doi.org/10.1177/1357034X04042938.

Dollar, David. 1998. "Macroeconomic Reform and Poverty Reduction in Vietnam." In *Household Welfare and Vietnam's Transition* (report). World Bank.

———. 2002. "Reform, Growth and Poverty in Vietnam." Development Research Group, World Bank.

Donaldson, Andrew. 2008. "Biosecurity after the Event: Risk Politics and Animal Disease." *Environment and Planning A* 40 (7): 1552–67. https://doi.org/10.1068/a4056.

Doreen, Thom van. 2014. "Care." *The Multispecies Salon* (blog). http://www.multispecies-salon .org/care/. Accessed June 6, 2018.

Douglas, Mary. 1992. *Risk and Blame: Essays in Cultural Theory.* London: Routledge.

Drummond, Lisa Barbara Welch, and Helle Rydstrøm. 2004. *Gender Practices in Contemporary Vietnam.* Singapore: National University of Singapore Press.

Duc, N. V., and T. Long. 2008. "Poultry Production Systems in Vietnam." GCP/RAS/228/GER Working Paper No. 4. Rome: Food and Agriculture Organization of the United Nations. http://www.fao.org/docrep/013/al693e/al693e00.pdf. Accessed May 17, 2015.

Dunn, Elizabeth C. 2005. "Standards and Person-Making in East Central Europe." In *Global Assemblages: Technology, Politics, and Ethics as Anthropological Problems.* Malden, MA: Blackwell.

Dutta, Mohan J. 2015. *Neoliberal Health Organizing: Communication, Meaning, and Politics.* Walnut Creek, CA: Routledge.

Enticott, Gareth. 2008. "The Spaces of Biosecurity: Prescribing and Negotiating Solutions to Bovine Tuberculosis." *Environment and Planning A* 40 (7): 1568–82. https://doi.org/10.1068/ a40304.

Evans-Pritchard, E. E. 1940. *The Nuer.* Oxford: Oxford University Press.

———. 1976. *Witchcraft, Oracles and Magic among the Azande.* Oxford: Oxford University Press.

Farmer, Paul. 2011. *Haiti after the Earthquake.* Philadelphia: PublicAffairs.

Farquhar, Judith, and Margaret Lock, eds. 2007. *Beyond the Body Proper: Reading the Anthropology of Material Life.* Durham, NC: Duke University Press.

Fearnley, Lyle. 2015. "Wild Goose Chase: The Displacement of Influenza Research in the Fields of Poyang Lake, China." *Cultural Anthropology* 30 (1): 12–35. https://doi.org/10.14506/ca30 .1.03.

———. 2018. "After the Livestock Revolution: Free-Grazing Ducks and Influenza Uncertainties in South China." *Medicine Anthropology Theory: An Open-Access Journal in the Anthropology of Health, Illness, and Medicine* 5 (3): 72. https://doi.org/10.17157/mat.5.3.378.

Fermet-Quinet, E., M. Edan, and J. Stratton. 2010. "Tool for the Evaluation of Performance of Veterinary Services." World Organization for Animal Health. http://www.oie.int/ fileadmin/Home/eng/Support_to_OIE_Members/pdf/A_PVS_Tool_Final_Edition_2013 .pdf. Accessed October 23, 2013.

Fermet-Quinet, E., R. Jane, and S. Forman. 2007. "Performance, Vision and Strategy: A Tool for the Governance of Veterinary Services." World Organization for Animal Health. http://

www.oie.int/fileadmin/Home/eng/Support_to_OIE_Members/docs/pdf/Brazil_OIE
-PVS-final_261207.pdf. Accessed November 3, 2013.

Fforde, Adam. 2005. "Vietnam in 2004: Popular Authority Seeking Power?" *Asian Survey* 45 (1): 146–52.

Fidler, David. 2008. "Influenza Virus Samples, International Law, and Global Health Diplomacy." *Emerging Infectious Diseases* 14 (1): 88–94.

Fischer, Michael M. J. 2005. "Technoscientific Infrastructures and Emergent Forms of Life: A Commentary." *American Anthropologist* 107 (1): 55–61.

Food and Agriculture Organization, World Health Organization, and World Organization for Animal Health. 2010. "The FAO-OIE-WHO Collaboration: Sharing Responsibilities and Coordinating Global Activities to Address Health Risks at the Animal-Human-Ecosystems Interfaces." OIE. http://web.oie.int/downld/FINAL_CONCEPT_NOTE_Hanoi.pdf. Accessed Februrary 4, 2012.

Fortun, Michæl A. 2008. *Promising Genomics: Iceland and DeCODE Genetics in a World of Speculation*. Oakland: University of California Press.

Fortun, Kim, and Mike Fortun. 2005. "Scientific Imaginaries and Ethical Plateaus in Contemporary U.S. Toxicology." *American Anthropologist* 107 (1): 43–54.

Foucault, Michel. 1991. "Governmentality." In *The Foucault Effect: Studies in Governmentality: With Two Lectures by and an Interview with Michel Foucault*, 87–104. Chicago: University of Chicago Press.

Franklin, Sarah. 2007. *Dolly Mixtures: The Remaking of Genealogy*. Durham, NC: Duke University Press.

Fritzen, Scott A. 2007. "Legacies of Primary Health Care in an Age of Health Sector Reform: Vietnam's Commune Clinics in Transition." *Social Science & Medicine* 64 (8): 1611–23. https://doi.org/10.1016/j.socscimed.2006.12.008.

Gainsborough, Martin. 1997. "Political Change in Vietnam." In *Democratization*, edited by D. Potter, D. Goldblatt, M. Kiloh, and P. Lewis, 490–512. Cambridge: Polity.

———. 2010. "Present but Not Powerful: Neoliberalism, the State, and Development in Vietnam." *Globalizations* 7 (4): 475–88. https://doi.org/10.1080/14747731003798435.

Gammeltoft, Tine. 1998. *Women's Bodies, Women's Worries: Health and Family Planning in a Vietnamese Rural Commune*. Abingdon, UK: Routledge.

———. 2008. "Childhood Disability and Parental Moral Responsibility in Northern Vietnam: Towards Ethnographies of Intercorporeality." *Journal of the Royal Anthropological Institute* 14 (4): 825–42.

Garrett, Laurie. 2015. "Ebola's Lessons." *Foreign Affairs*, December 11. https://www.foreignaffairs.com/articles/west-africa/2015-08-18/ebolas-lessons. Accessed March 2, 2016.

Gauthier-Clerc, M., C. Lebarbenchon, and F. Thomas. 2007. "Recent Expansion of Highly Pathogenic Avian Influenza H5N1: A Critical Review." *International Journal of Avian Science* 149 (2): 202–14.

Geissler, Paul Wenzel. 2015. "Introduction: A Life Science in Its African Para-State." In *Para-States and Medical Science: Making African Global Health*, edited by Paul Wenzel Geissler, 1–46. Durham, NC: Duke University Press.

Geissler, Paul Wenzel, and Ann H. Kelly. 2016. "Field Station as Stage: Re-Enacting Scientific Work and Life in Amani, Tanzania." *Social Studies of Science* 46 (6): 912–37. https://doi.org/10.1177/0306312716650045.

Gilbert, M., X. Xiao, D. U. Pfeiffer, M. Epprecht, S. Boles, C. Czarnecki, P. Chaitaweesub, et al.

2008. "Mapping H5N1 Highly Pathogenic Avian Influenza Risk in Southeast Asia." *Proceedings of the National Academy of Sciences* 105 (12): 4769–74. https://doi.org/10.1073/pnas .0710581105.

Giraud, Eva, and Gregory Hollin. 2016. "Care, Laboratory Beagles and Affective Utopia." *Theory, Culture & Society* (January), 0263276415619685. https://doi.org/10.1177/0263276415619685.

Goscha, Christopher. 2016. *Vietnam: A New History.* New York: Basic Books.

Graeber, David. 2001. *Toward an Anthropological Theory of Value: The False Coin of Our Own Dreams.* 1st ed. New York: Palgrave Macmillan.

Greenhough, Beth. 2012. "Where Species Meet and Mingle: Endemic Human-Virus Relations, Embodied Communication and More-than-Human Agency at the Common Cold Unit 1946–90." *Cultural Geographies* 19 (3): 281–301. https://doi.org/10.1177/1474474011422029.

Greenhough, Beth, and Emma Roe. 2011. "Ethics, Space, and Somatic Sensibilities: Comparing Relationships between Scientific Researchers and Their Human and Animal Experimental Subjects." *Environment and Planning D: Society and Space* 29 (1): 47–66. https://doi.org/10 .1068/d17109.

Gruen, Lori. 2014. *Entangled Empathy: An Alternative Ethic for Our Relationships with Animals.* New York: Lantern.

Guerrero Blanco, Tomas. 2013. "Frontier Markets: A World of Opportunities." SSRN Scholarly Paper ID 2245075. Rochester, NY: Social Science Research Network. http://papers.ssrn .com/abstract=2245075.

Hallowell, Alfred Irving. 1992. *The Ojibwa of Berens River, Manitoba: Ethnography Into History.* San Diego, CA: Harcourt Brace Jovanovich.

Haraway, Donna. 2007. *When Species Meet.* Minneapolis: University of Minnesota Press.

Harms, Erik. 2011. *Saigon's Edge: On the Margins of Ho Chi Minh City.* Minneapolis: University of Minnesota Press.

Harris, Marvin. 1974. *Cows, Pigs, Wars and Witches: The Riddles of Culture.* New York: Random House.

Hartigan, John. 2014. *Aesop's Anthropology: A Multispecies Approach.* Minneapolis: University of Minnesota Press.

———. 2015. "Ethnography of Life Forms." *Engagement* (blog). September 8. https://aesengage ment.wordpress.com/2015/09/08/ethnography-of-life-forms/. Accessed March 2, 2018.

Harvie, Charles. 1997. *Vietnam's Reforms and Economic Growth.* New York: St. Martin's Press.

Hayden, Cori. 2003. *When Nature Goes Public: The Making and Unmaking of Bioprospecting in Mexico.* Princeton, NJ: Princeton University Press.

Heather, David, and Sherry Buchanan. 2009. *Vietnam Posters: The David Heather Collection.* Munich: Prestel.

Helmreich, Stefan. 2009. *Alien Ocean: Anthropological Voyages in Microbial Seas.* Oakland: University of California Press.

Helmreich, Stefan, and Sophia Roosth. 2016. "Life Forms: A Keyword Entry." In *Sounding the Limits of Life: Essays in the Anthropology of Biology and Beyond*, by Stefan Helmreich, Sophia Roosth, and Michelle Friedner, 19–34. Princeton, NJ: Princeton University Press.

Hilgartner, Stephen. 2013. "Constituting Large-Scale Biology: Building a Regime of Governance in the Early Years of the Human Genome Project." *BioSocieties* 8 (4): 397–416. https://doi .org/10.1057/biosoc.2013.31.

Hinchliffe, Steve. 2001. "Indeterminacy In-Decisions: Science, Policy and Politics in the BSE (Bovine Spongiform Encephalopathy) Crisis." *Transactions of the Institute of British Geographers*, n.s., 26 (2): 182–204.

Hinchliffe, Steve, and Nick Bingham. 2008. "Securing Life: The Emerging Practices of Bio-security." *Environment and Planning A* 40 (7): 1534–51. https://doi.org/10.1068/a4054.

Hinchliffe, Steve, Gareth Enticott, and Nick Bingham. 2008. "Biosecurity: Spaces, Practices, and Boundaries." *Environment and Planning A* 40: 1528–33.

Hinterberger, Amy, and Natalie Porter. 2015. "Genomic and Viral Sovereignty: Tethering the Materials of Global Biomedicine." *Public Culture* 27 (2 (76)): 361–86. https://doi.org/10.1215/08992363-2841904.

Ho Chi Minh. 2001. *Ho Chi Minh: Selected Writings 1920–1969*. Honolulu, HI: University Press of the Pacific.

Holbrooke, Richard, and Laurie Garrett. 2008. "'Sovereignty' that Risks Global Health." *Washington Post*, 2008, sec. Opinions. http://www.washingtonpost.com/wp-dyn/content/article/2008/08/08/AR2008080802919.html. Accessed March 2, 2012.

Hong Hanh, P. T. H., S. Burgos, and D. Roland-Holst. 2007. "The Poultry Sector in Viet Nam: Prospects for Smallholder Producers in the Aftermath of the HPAI Crisis." Research report. Pro-Poor Livestock Policy Initiative Research Report. Rome: Food and Agricultural Organization of the United Nations. http://agris.fao.org/agris-search/search.do?recordID=XF2006446597. Accessed March 12, 2012.

Honhold, Nick, Annie McLeod, Satyajit Sarkar, and Phil Harris. 2008. "Biosecurity for Highly Pathogenic Avian Influenza: Issues and Options." Rome: Food and Agriculture Organization of the United Nations. http://www.fao.org/3/a-i0359e.pdf. Accessed October 8, 2013.

Horowitz, Roger. 2004. "Making the Chicken of Tomorrow: Reworking Poultry as Commodities and as Creatures, 1945–1990." In *Industrialising Organisms: Introducing Evolutionary History*, edited by Susan R. Schrepfer and Philip Scranton, 215–36. New York: Routledge.

Hutchinson, Sharon. 1996. *Nuer Dilemmas: Coping with Money, War, and the State*. Oakland: University of California Press.

———. 1992. "The Cattle of Money and the Cattle of Girls among the Nuer, 1930–83." *American Ethnologist* 19 (2): 294–316.

Ifft, J., J. Otte, D. Roland-Holst, Nguyen Do Anh Tuan, and Nguyen Duc Loc. 2010. "Safety Certified Free-Range Duck Supply Chains Enhance Both Public Health and Livelihoods." http://r4d.dfid.gov.uk/Output/183551/Default.aspx. Accessed July 2, 2013.

Ingold, Tim. 1980. *Hunters, Pastoralists, and Ranchers: Reindeer Economies and Their Transformations*. Cambridge: Cambridge University Press.

———. 1988. *What Is an Animal?* London: Unwin Hyman.

International Committee of the OIE. 2008. "Resolution No XXVI: Sharing of Avian Influenza Viral Material and Information in Support of Global Avian Influenza Prevention and Control." Paris. http://wahis2-devt.oie.int/doc/ged/D4841.PDF. Accessed June 23, 2018.

Jamieson, Neil L. 1995. *Understanding Vietnam*. Oakland: University of California Press.

Janes, Craig R., and Kitty K. Corbett. 2009. "Anthropology and Global Health." *Annual Review of Anthropology* 38: 167–83.

Justino, Patricia, Julie Litchfield, and Hung Thai Pham. 2008. "Poverty Dynamics During Trade Reform: Evidence from Rural Vietnam." *Review of Income and Wealth* 54 (2): 166–92. https://doi.org/10.1111/j.1475-4991.2008.00269.x.

Keck, Frédéric. 2008. "From Mad Cow Disease to Bird Flu: Transformations of Food Safety in France." In *Biosecurity Interventions: Global Health and Security in Question*, edited by Andrew Lakoff and Stephen J. Collier, 195–227. New York: Columbia University Press.

———. 2014. "Birds as Sentinels for Pandemic Influenza." *BioSocieties* 9 (2): 223–25. https://doi.org/10.1057/biosoc.2014.9.

―――. 2015. "Feeding Sentinels: Logics of Care and Biosecurity in Farms and Labs." *Bio-Societies* 10 (2): 162–76. https://doi.org/10.1057/biosoc.2015.6.

―――. 2016. "Storage and Stockpiling as Techniques of Preparedness: Managing the Bottle-necks of Flu Pandemics; Somatosphere." *Somatosphere: Science, Medicine, and Anthropology* (blog). http://somatosphere.net/2016/06/storage-and-stockpiling-as-techniques-of-preparedness-managing-the-bottlenecks-of-flu-pandemics.html. Accessed July 16, 2018.

Keevers, Lynne, Lesley Treleaven, and Chris Sykes. 2008. "Partnership and Participation: Con-tradictions and Tensions in the Social Policy Space." *Australian Journal of Social Issues* 43 (3): 459–77.

Kelly, Ann H., and Javier Lezaun. 2013. "Walking or Waiting? Topologies of the Breeding Ground in Malaria Control." *Science as Culture* 22 (1): 86–107. https://doi.org/10.1080/09505431.2013.776368.

Khor, Martin. 2007. "Indonesia to Share Bird-Flu Samples Only If There Is New System: Our World Is Not for Sale." February 22, 2007. http://www.ourworldisnotforsale.org/es/node/1983. Accessed June 2, 2015.

Kipnis, Andrew. 2007. "Neoliberalism Reified: Suzhi Discourse and Tropes of Neoliberalism in the People's Republic of China." *Journal of the Royal Anthropological Institute* 13 (2): 383–400. https://doi.org/10.1111/j.1467-9655.2007.00432.x.

―――. 2008. "Audit Cultures: Neoliberal Governmentality, Socialist Legacy, or Technologies of Governing?" *American Ethnologist* 35 (2): 275–89. https://doi.org/10.1111/j.1548-1425.2008.00034.x.

Kirksey, Eben, ed. 2014. *The Multispecies Salon.* Durham, NC: Duke University Press.

Kirksey, S. Eben, and Stefan Helmreich. 2010. "The Emergence of Multispecies Ethnography." *Cultural Anthropology* 25 (4): 545–76. https://doi.org/10.1111/j.1548-1360.2010.01069.x.

Koch, Erin. 2013. *Free Market Tuberculosis: Managing Epidemics in Post-Soviet Georgia.* Nash-ville, TN: Vanderbilt University Press.

Kohler, Robert E. 1994. *Lords of the Fly: Drosophila Genetics and the Experimental Life.* Chicago: University of Chicago Press.

Kohn, Eduardo. 2013. *How Forests Think: Toward an Anthropology Beyond the Human.* Oakland: University of California Press.

Lakoff, Andrew. 2007. "Preparing for the Next Emergency." *Public Culture* 19 (2): 247–71. https://doi.org/10.1215/08992363-2006-035.

―――. 2010. "Two Regimes of Global Health." *Humanity: An International Journal of Human Rights, Humanitarianism and Development* 1 (1): 57–59.

―――. 2017. *Unprepared: Global Health in a Time of Emergency.* 1st ed. Oakland: University of California Press.

Latimer, Joanna. 2013. "Being Alongside: Rethinking Relations amongst Different Kinds." *The-ory, Culture & Society* 30 (7–8): 77–104. https://doi.org/10.1177/0263276413500078.

Le, Thomas. 2005. "Vietnamese Poetry." *The Huu Van Dan: The Literary Forum* (blog). http://thehuuvandan.org/vietpoet.html. Accessed June 23, 2018.

Leaf, Michael L. 1999. *Urbanization on the Periphery: A Hanoi Case Study.* Vancouver: University of British Columbia.

Leibler, Jessica, Joachim Otte, David Roland-Holst, Dirk Pfeiffer, Ricardo Magalhaes, Jonathan Rushton, Jay Graham, and Ellen Silbergeld. 2009. "Industrial Food Animal Production and Global Health Risks: Exploring the Ecosystems and Economics of Avian Influenza." *Eco-Health* March 6 (1): 58–70.

Leonardi, Paul M. 2010. "Digital Materiality? How Artifacts without Matter, Matter." *First Monday* 15 (6–7). http://firstmonday.org/ojs/index.php/fm/article/view/3036. Accessed July 3, 2018.

Leonelli, Sabina. 2016. *Data-Centric Biology: A Philosophical Study.* Chicago: University of Chicago Press.

Leonelli, Sabina, and Rachel A. Ankeny. 2013. "What Makes a Model Organism?" *Endeavour* 37 (4): 209–12. https://doi.org/10.1016/j.endeavour.2013.06.001.

Leshkowich, Ann Marie. 2012. "Rendering Infant Abandonment Technical and Moral: Expertise, Neoliberal Logics, and Class Differentiation in Ho Chi Minh City." *Positions: East Asia Cultures Critique* 20 (2): 497–526.

———. 2014. "Standardized Forms of Vietnamese Selfhood: An Ethnographic Genealogy of Documentation." *American Ethnologist* 41 (1): 143–62. https://doi.org/10.1111/amet.12065.

Lezaun, Javier, and Catherine M. Montgomery. 2015. "The Pharmaceutical Commons Sharing and Exclusion in Global Health Drug Development." *Science, Technology & Human Values* 40 (1): 3–29. https://doi.org/10.1177/0162243914542349.

Lezaun, Javier, and Natalie Porter. 2015. "Containment and Competition: Transgenic Animals in the One Health Agenda." *Social Science & Medicine* 129 (March): 96–105. https://doi.org/10.1016/j.socscimed.2014.06.024.

Li, Tania Murray. 2007. *The Will to Improve: Governmentality, Development, and the Practice of Politics.* Durham, NC: Duke University Press.

———. 2014. *Land's End: Capitalist Relations on an Indigenous Frontier.* Durham, NC: Duke University Press.

Lien, Marianne Elisabeth. 2015. *Becoming Salmon: Aquaculture and the Domestication of a Fish.* Oakland: University of California Press.

Liljeström, Rita, Van Ang Nguyen, Eva Lindskog, and Xuan Tinh Vuong. 1998. *Profit and Poverty in Rural Vietnam: Winners and Losers of a Dismantled Revolution.* Surrey, UK: Curzon.

Liu, Qinfang, Ignacio Mena, Jingjiao Ma, Bhupinder Bawa, Florian Krammer, Young S. Lyoo, Yuekun Lang, et al. 2015. "Newcastle Disease Virus-Vectored H7 and H5 Live Vaccines Protect Chickens from Challenge with H7N9 or H5N1 Avian Influenza Viruses." *Journal of Virology* (April), JVI.00031-15. https://doi.org/10.1128/JVI.00031-15.

Lorimer, Jamie. 2017. "Parasites, Ghosts and Mutualists: A Relational Geography of Microbes for Global Health." *Transactions of the Institute of British Geographers* 42 (4): 544–58. https://doi.org/10.1111/tran.12189.

———. 2018. "Hookworms Make Us Human: The Microbiome, Eco-Immunology, and a Probiotic Turn in Western Health Care." *Medical Anthropology Quarterly* advance online publication (ja). https://doi.org/10.1111/maq.12466.

Lowe, Celia. 2006. *Wild Profusion: Biodiversity Conservation in an Indonesian Archipelago.* Princeton, NJ: Princeton University Press.

———. 2010. "Viral Clouds: Becoming H5N1 in Indonesia." *Cultural Anthropology* 25 (4): 625–49. https://doi.org/10.1111/j.1548-1360.2010.01072.x.

Lupton, Deborah. 2016. "Digital Companion Species and Eating Data: Implications for Theorising Digital Data–Human Assemblages." *Big Data & Society* 3 (1): 1–5. https://doi.org/10.1177/2053951715619947.

Luong, Hy Van. 2006. "Structure, Practice, and History: Contemporary Anthropological Research on Vietnam." *Journal of Vietnamese Studies* 1 (1–2): 371–409.

Luong, Hy Van, ed. 2003. *Postwar Vietnam: Dynamics of a Transforming Society.* Singapore: Rowman & Littlefield.

Mabbett, Terry. 2009. "H5N1 Sample Hoarding Begins to Backfire on Indonesia's Poultry Industry." WATTAgNet: News and Analysis on the Global Poultry and Animal Feed Industries. June 30. https://www.wattagnet.com/articles/670-h5n1-sample-hoarding-begins-to
-backfire-on-indonesia. Accessed June 5, 2017.

MacKenzie, Debora. 2015. "US Farms Hit by Bird Flu—but a Vaccine Might Make Things
Worse." *New Scientist* (blog), April. https://www.newscientist.com/article/dn27423-us
-farms-hit-by-bird-flu-but-a-vaccine-might-make-things-worse/. Accessed June 5, 2017.

MacPhail, Theresa. 2004. "The Viral Gene: An Undead Metaphor Recoding Life." *Science as
Culture* 13 (3): 325–45. https://doi.org/10.1080/0950543042000262413.

———. 2014a. "Limn: Global Health Doesn't Exist." *Limn.* December 19. https://limn.it/
articles/global-health-doesnt-exist/.

———. 2014b. *The Viral Network: A Pathography of the H1N1 Influenza Pandemic.* Ithaca, NY:
Cornell University Press.

Malarney, Shaun Kingsley. 1996. "The Limits of 'State Functionalism' and the Reconstruction of
Funerary Ritual in Contemporary Northern Vietnam." *American Ethnologist* 23 (3): 540–
60. https://doi.org/10.1525/ae.1996.23.3.02a00050.

———. 2012. "Germ Theory, Hygiene and the Transcendence of 'Backwardness' in Revolutionary Vietnam (1954–60)." In *Southern Medicine for Southern People: Vietnamese Medicine in
the Making,* edited by Laurence Monnais, Michelle Thompson, and Ayo Wahlberg, 107–32.
Newcastle upon Tyne, UK: Cambridge Scholars Publishing.

Marcus, George, and Michael Fischer. 1999. *Anthropology as Cultural Critique: An Experimental Moment in the Human Sciences by George E. Marcus.* Chicago: University of Chicago
Press.

Marr, David G. 1981. *Vietnamese Tradition on Trial, 1920–1945.* Berkeley: University of California
Press.

McKenna, Maryn. 2006. "Vietnam's Success Against Avian Flu May Offer Blueprint for Others."
Special Report on Bird Flu in Vietnam. Pt. 1. Minneapolis: University of Minnesota. http://
www.cidrap.umn.edu. Accessed November 7, 2011.

Mcleod, A., O. Thieme, and S. D. Mack. 2009. "Structural Changes in the Poultry Sector: Will
There Be Smallholder Poultry Development in 2030?" *World's Poultry Science Journal* 65 (2):
191–200. https://doi.org/10.1017/S0043933909000129.

McLeod, Annie, Nancy Morgan, Adam Prakash, and Jan Hinrichs. 2006. "Economic and Social Impacts of Avian Influenza." Rome: Food and Agriculture Organization of the United
Nations.   http://www.fao.org/docs/eims/upload//211939/Economic-and-social-impacts
-of-avian-influenza-Geneva.pdf. Accessed May 18, 2018.

Ministry of Health, and Ministry of Agriculture and Rural Development. 2010. "Avian and Pandemic Influenza: Vietnam's Experience." Hanoi: Interministerial Conference on Animal
and Pandemic Influenza (IMCAPI).

Mol, Annemarie. 2008. *The Logic of Care: Health and the Problem of Patient Choice.* New York:
Routledge.

Montoya, Alfred. 2012. "From 'the People' to 'the Human': HIV/AIDS, Neoliberalism, and the
Economy of Virtue in Contemporary Vietnam." *Positions: East Asia Cultures Critique* 20
(2): 561–91.

Morris, R., R. Jackson, M. Stevenson, J. Bernard, and N. Cogger. 2005. "Epidemiology of H5N1
Avian Influenza in Asia and Implications for Regional Control." Rome: Food and Agriculture Organization of the United Nations. http://www.fao.org/docs/eims/upload/246974/
aj122e00.pdf. Accessed September 6, 2013.

Muñoz, José Esteban. 2015. "Theorizing Queer Inhumanisms: The Sense of Brownness." *GLQ: A Journal of Lesbian and Gay Studies* 21 (2): 209–10.

Murphy, Michelle. 2017. *The Economization of Life*. Durham, NC: Duke University Press.

Nadasdy, Paul. 2003. *Hunters and Bureaucrats: Power, Knowledge, and Aboriginal-State Relations in the Southwest Yukon*. Vancouver: University of British Columbia Press.

———. 2007. "The Gift in the Animal: The Ontology of Hunting and Human-Animal Sociality." *American Ethnologist* 34 (1): 25–43.

Nading, Alex M. 2014a. "The Lively Ethics of Global Health GMOs: The Case of the Oxitec Mosquito." *BioSocieties* (June). https://doi.org/10.1057/biosoc.2014.16.

———. 2014b. *Mosquito Trails: Ecology, Health, and the Politics of Entanglement*. 1st ed. Oakland: University of California Press.

———. 2016. "Evidentiary Symbiosis: On Paraethnography in Human–Microbe Relations." *Science as Culture* 25 (4): 560–81. https://doi.org/10.1080/09505431.2016.1202226.

National Steering Committee on Avian and Human Influenza. 2006a. *Partnership Agreement between the National Steering Committee for Avian Influenza of the Socialist Republic of Vietnam and International Partners: Concerning the Establishment of the Vietnam Partnership on Avian and Human Pandemic Influenza (PAHI)*. Hanoi: Socialist Republic of Vietnam.

———. 2006b. *Vietnam Integrated National Plan for Avian Influenza Control and Human Pandemic Influenza Response 2006–2008*. Hanoi: Socialist Republic of Vietnam.

———. 2006c. "Vietnam Integrated National Operational Program for Avian and Human Influenza (OPI) 2006–2010." Hanoi: Socialist Republic of Vietnam.

———. 2008. "National Strategic Framework for Avian and Human Influenza Communications 2008–2010." Hanoi: Partnership for Avian and Human Influenza.

Nelson, Nicole C. 2013. "Modeling Mouse, Human, and Discipline: Epistemic Scaffolds in Animal Behavior Genetics." *Social Studies of Science* 43 (1): 3–29. https://doi.org/10.1177/0306312712463815.

———. 2018. *Model Behavior: Animal Experiments, Complexity, and the Genetics of Psychiatric Disorders*. Chicago: University of Chicago Press. https://www.press.uchicago.edu/ucp/books/book/chicago/M/bo27949249.html.

Nguyen, Bich Thuan, Curt Lofgren, Lars Lindholm, and Nguyen T. K. Chuc. 2008. "Choice of Healthcare Provider Following Reform in Vietnam." *BMC Health Services Research* 8 (1): 162. https://doi.org/10.1186/1472-6963-8-162.

Nguyen, Bich Thuan, and Mandy Thomas. 2004. "Young Women and Emergent Postsocialist Sensibilities in Contemporary Vietnam." *Asian Studies Review* 28 (2): 133–49.

Nguyen, Van Suu. 2004. "The Politics of Land: Inequality in Land Access and Local Conflicts in the Red River Delta since Decollectivization." In *Social Inequality in Vietnam and the Challenges to Reform*, edited by Philip Taylor, 270–96. Singapore: Institute of Southeast Asian Studies.

Nguyen, Vinh Kim. 2005. "Antiretroviral Globalism, Biopolitics, and Therapeutic Citizenship." In *Global Assemblages: Technology, Politics and Ethics as Anthropological Problems*, 124–44. Malden, MA: Blackwell.

———. 2009. "Government-by-Exception: Enrollment and Experimentality in Mass HIV Treatment Programmes in Africa." *Social Theory & Health* 7 (3): 196–217. https://doi.org/10.1057/sth.2009.12.

———. 2015. "Treating to Prevent HIV: Population Trials and Experimental Societies." In *Para-States and Medical Science: Making African Global Health*, edited by Paul Wenzel Geissler, 47–77. Durham, NC: Duke University Press.

Nguyen-Marshall, Van, Lisa B. Welch Drummond, and Danièle Bélanger. 2011. *The Reinvention of Distinction: Modernity and the Middle Class in Urban Vietnam*. London: Springer.

Nguyen-Vo, Thu-Huong. 2008. *The Ironies of Freedom: Sex, Culture, and Neoliberal Governance in Vietnam*. Seattle: University of Washington Press.

Novas, Carlos, and Nikolas Rose. 2005. "Biological Citizenship." In *Global Assemblages: Technology, Politics and Ethics as Anthropological Problems*. Edited by Aihwa Ong and Stephen Collier, 439–463. Malden, MA: Blackwell.

Novelli, W. 1990. "Applying Social Marketing to Health Promotion and Disease Prevention." In *Health Behavior and Health Education: Theory, Research and Practice*, edited by K. Glanz, F. M. Lewis, and B. K. Rimer, 324–69. San Francisco: Jossey-Bass.

OFFLU. 2018. "Mission and Objectives: OFFLU's Vision." OFFLU: Network of Expertise on Animal Influenza. http://www.offlu.net/index.php?id=52. Accessed March 2, 2018.

———. 2018. "OFFLU Position on Material Transfer Agreements." OFFLU OIE/FAO Network of Expertise on Animal Influenza: OFFLU Statement on MTA. http://www.offlu.net/index.php?id=169. Accessed March 12, 2018.

Ogden, Laura A. 2011. *Swamplife: People, Gators, and Mangroves Entangled in the Everglades*. Minneapolis: University of Minnesota Press.

Ogden, Laura A., Billy Hall, and Kimiko Tanita. 2013. "Animals, Plants, People, and Things: A Review of Multispecies Ethnography." *Environment and Society* 4 (1): 5–24. https://doi.org/10.3167/ares.2013.040102.

Ong, Aihwa. 2006. *Neoliberalism as Exception: Mutations in Citizenship and Sovereignty*. Durham, NC: Duke University Press.

———. 2008. "Scales of Exception: Experiments with Knowledge and Sheer Life in Tropical Southeast Asia." *Singapore Journal of Tropical Geography* 29 (2): 117–129. https://doi.org/10.1111/j.1467-9493.2008.00323.x.

Otte, Joachim. 2007. "Smallholder Livestock Producers and Global Health Risk, Research Report PPLPI." Unpublished research report. Rome: Food and Agriculture Organization of the United Nations.

Otte, Joachim, David Roland-Holst, and Dirk Pfeiffer. 2006. "HPAI Control Measures and Household Incomes in Vietnam PPLPI." Rome: Food and Agriculture Organization of the United Nations. http://www.fao.org/docs/eims/upload/211942/Vietnam-HPAI_DRH.pdf. Accessed June 12, 2013.

Otte, Joachim, D. Pfeiffer, R. Soares-Magalhaes, S. Burgos, and D. Roland-Holst. 2008. "Flock Size and HPAI Risk in Cambodia, Thailand and Viet Nam." Research brief 5. Pro-Poor HPAI Risk Reduction Project. https://www.gov.uk/dfid-research-outputs/flock-size-and-hpai-risk-in-cambodia-thailand-and-viet-nam. Accessed July 30, 2018.

Pachirat, Timothy. 2013. *Every Twelve Seconds: Industrialized Slaughter and the Politics of Sight*. Yale Agrarian Studies series. New Haven, CT: Yale University Press.

Parrenas, Rheano "Juno" Salazar. 2012. "Producing Affect: Transnational Volunteerism in a Malaysian Orangutan Rehabilitation Center." *American Ethnologist* 39 (4): 673–87.

———. 2015. "Multispecies Ethnography and Social Hierarchy: Engagement." *Engagement: A Blog Published by the Anthropology Environment and Society*, September 15. https://aesengagement.wordpress.com/2015/09/15/multispecies-ethnography-and-social-hierarchy/. Accessed February 20, 2018.

Parry, Bronwyn. 2004. *Trading the Genome: Investigating the Commodification of Bio-Information*. New York: Columbia University Press.

Pashigian, Melissa J. 2012. "Counting One's Way onto the Global Stage: Enumeration, Account-ability, and Reproductive Success in Vietnam." *Positions: East Asia Cultures Critique* 20 (2): 529–58.

Paxson, Heather. 2008. "Post-Pasteurian Cultures: The Microbiopolitics of Raw-Milk Cheese in the United States." *Cultural Anthropology* 23 (1): 15–47. https://doi.org/10.1111/j.1548 -1360.2008.00002.x.

———. 2012. *The Life of Cheese: Crafting Food and Value in America.* Oakland: University of California Press.

Peckham, Robert, and David M. Pomfret, eds. 2013. *Imperial Contagions: Medicine, Hygiene, and Cultures of Planning in Asia.* Hong Kong: Hong Kong University Press.

Pelley, Patricia M. 2002. *Postcolonial Vietnam: New Histories of the National Past.* Durham, NC: Duke University Press.

Petryna, Adriana. 2002. *Life Exposed: Biological Citizens after Chernobyl.* Princeton, NJ: Princeton University Press.

———. 2009. *When Experiments Travel: Clinical Trials and the Global Search for Human Subjects.* Princeton, NJ: Princeton University Press.

Pettus, Ashley. 2003. *Between Sacrifice and Desire: National Identity and the Governing of Femininity in Vietnam.* New York: Routledge.

Peyre, M., S. Desvaux, G. Fusheng, and F. Roger. 2011. "Avian Influenza Vaccine Development, Practical Application in Developing Countries." CIRAD. avian-influenza.cirad.fr/content/ download/1727/ . . . /M_Peyre_AITVM.pdf. Accessed December 1, 2016.

Pfeiffer, James, and Mark Nichter. 2008. "What Can Critical Medical Anthropology Contribute to Global Health? A Health Systems Perspective." *Medical Anthropology Quarterly,* n.s., 22 (4): 410–15.

Pham, Thao, and David Roland-Holst. 2007. "Agro-Food Product Quality and Safety Management in Vietnam: An Overview of the Poultry Sector." Unpublished research report by the Pro-Poor Livestock Policy Initiative.

Phan, Thao. 2011. "Terminate Bird Flu Vaccine: Deputy Prime Minister." Translated by Phuong Uyen. *Sài Gòn Giải Phóng,* May 27, 2011, sec. Health. http://www.saigon-gpdaily.com.vn/ Health/2011/5/92987/.

Phuc, To Xuan. 2011. "When the Dai Gia (Urban Rich) Go to the Countryside: Impacts of the Urban-Fuelled Rural Land Market in the Uplands." In *The Reinvention of Distinction: Modernity and the Middle Class in Urban Vietnam,* edited by Van Nguyen-Marshall, Lisa B. Welch Drummond, and Danièle Bélanger, 143–56. New York: Springer.

Pink, Sarah, Elisenda Ardèvol, and Dèbora Lanzeni, eds. 2016. *Digital Materialities: Design and Anthropology.* London: Bloomsbury Academic.

Pink, Sarah, Minna Ruckenstein, Robert Willim, and Melisa Duque. 2018. "Broken Data: Conceptualising Data in an Emerging World." *Big Data & Society* 5 (1): 1–13. https://doi.org/10 .1177/2053951717753228.

Porter, Gareth. 1993. *The Politics of Bureaucratic Socialism.* Ithaca, NY: Cornell University Press.

———, ed. 1979. *Vietnam: The Definitive Documentation of Human Decisions.* Vol. 2. Stanfordville, NY: Earl M. Coleman Enterprises, Inc.

Porter, Natalie. 2013. "Bird Flu Biopower: Strategies for Multispecies Coexistence in Việt Nam." *American Ethnologist* 40 (1): 132–48. https://doi.org/10.1111/amet.12010.

———. 2015. "Ferreting Things Out: Biosecurity, Pandemic Flu and the Transformation of Experimental Systems." *BioSocieties* (March). https://doi.org/10.1057/biosoc.2015.4.

———. 2018. "Read, Respond, Rescue." In *Living with Animals: Bonds across Species*, edited by Natalie Porter and Ilana Gershon, 223–35. Ithaca, NY: Cornell University Press.

Povinelli, Elizabeth A. 1995. "Do Rocks Listen? The Cultural Politics of Apprehending Australian Aboriginal Labor." *American Anthropologist* 97 (3): 505–18.

PricewaterhouseCoopers. 2017. "The Long View: How Will the Global Economic Order Change by 2050?" https://www.pwc.com/gx/en/world-2050/assets/pwc-the-world-in-2050-full -report-feb-2017.pdf. Accessed July 25, 2018.

Pritchett, Lant. 1993. "A Toy Collection, a Socialist Star, and a Democratic Dud? Growth Theory, Vietnam and the Philippines." In *In Search of Prosperity: Analytic Narratives on Economic Growth*, edited by Dani Rodrick. Princeton, NJ: Princeton University Press.

ProMED. 2011. "Avian Influenza- MBDS Region (08): Viet Nam." RF. *ProMED-Mail, International Society for Infectious Diseases.* http://www.promedmail.org/post/20110531.1662. Accessed February 24, 2012.

Rader, Karen Ann. 2004. *Making Mice: Standardizing Animals for American Biomedical Research, 1900–1955.* Princeton, NJ: Princeton University Press.

Rappaport, Roy A. 1967. *Pigs for the Ancestors: Ritual in the Ecology of a New Guinea People.* New Haven, CT: Yale University Press.

Reynolds Whyte, Susan, Michael Whyte, Lotte Meinert, and Jenipher Twebaze. 2013. "Therapeutic Clientship." In *When People Come First: Critical Studies in Global Health*, edited by Joao Biehl and Adriana Petryna, 140–65. Princeton, NJ: Princeton University Press.

Rheinberger, Hans-Jorg. 1997. *Toward a History of Epistemic Things: Synthesizing Proteins in the Test Tube (Writing Science).* Palo Alto, CA: Stanford University Press.

Ritvo, Harriet. 1987. *The Animal Estate: The English and Other Creatures in the Victorian Age.* Cambridge, MA: Harvard University Press.

R. J. 2018. "What Is Disease X?" *The Economist*, March 23. https://www.economist.com/the -economist-explains/2018/03/23/what-is-disease-x. Accessed April 20, 2018.

Rock, Melanie J., and Chris Degeling. 2015. "Public Health Ethics and More-than-Human Solidarity." *Social Science & Medicine (1982)* 129 (March): 61–67. https://doi.org/10.1016/j .socscimed.2014.05.050.

Rofel, Lisa. 2007. *Desiring China: Experiments in Neoliberalism, Sexuality, and Public Culture.* Durham, NC: Duke University Press.

Rogaski, Ruth. 2004. *Hygienic Modernity: Meanings of Health and Disease in Treaty-Port China.* Oakland: University of California Press.

Rose, Nikolas. 2006. *The Politics of Life Itself: Biomedicine, Power, and Subjectivity in the Twenty-First Century.* Princeton, NJ: Princeton University Press.

Rota, Antonio, and Sylvia Sperandini. 2010. "Value Chains, Linking Producers to the Markets." Livestock Thematic Papers Tools for Project Design. Rome: International Fund for Agricultural Development. https://www.slideshare.net/copppldsecretariat/value-chains -15766121. Accessed July 30, 2018.

Rottenburg, Richard. 2009. "Social and Public Experiments and New Figurations of Science and Politics in Postcolonial Africa." *Postcolonial Studies* 12 (4): 423–40. https://doi.org/10.1080/ 13688790903350666.

Salemink, Oscar. 2003. "One Country, Many Journeys." In *Vietnam: Journeys of Body, Mind and Spirit*, edited by Nguyen Van Huy and Laurel Kendall, 20–51. Oakland: University of California Press.

———. 2006. "Translating, Interpreting and Practicing Civil Society in Vietnam: A Tale of Calculated Misunderstandings." In *Development Brokers and Translators: The Ethnography of Aid and Agencies*, edited by David Lewis and David Mosse, 101–26. Bloomfield, CT: Kumarian Press.

Samimian-Darash, Limor. 2009. "A Pre-Event Configuration for Biological Threats: Preparedness and the Constitution of Biosecurity Events." *American Ethnologist* 36 (3): 478–91. https://doi.org/10.1111/j.1548-1425.2009.01174.x.

Samsky, Ari. 2012. "Scientific Sovereignty: How International Drug Donation Programs Reshape Health, Disease, and the State." *Cultural Anthropology* 27 (2): 310–32. https://doi.org/10.1111/j.1548-1360.2012.01145.x.

Scheper-Hughes, Nancy, and Margaret Lock. 1987. "The Mindful Body: A Prolegomenon to Future Work in Medical Anthropology." *Medical Anthropology Quarterly* 1 (March): 6–41.

Schwenkel, Christina, and Ann Marie Leshkowich. 2012. "Guest Editors' Introduction: How Is Neoliberalism Good to Think Vietnam? How Is Vietnam Good to Think Neoliberalism?" *Positions: Asia Critique* 20 (2): 379–401. https://doi.org/10.1215/10679847-1538461.

Scott, James C. 1976. *The Moral Economy of the Peasant: Rebellion and Subsistence in Southeast Asia*. New Haven, CT: Yale University Press.

Sedyaningsih, Endand, Siti Isfandari, Triono Soendro, and Siti Fadilah Supari. 2008. "Towards Mutual Trust, Transparency and Equity in Virus Sharing Mechanism: The Avian Influenza Case of Indonesia." *Annals of the Academy of Medicine* 37 (6): 482–88.

Sepheri, A., and A. H. Akram-Lodhi. 2005. "Adjustment, Transition and the Provision of Health Care: Vietnam's Experience." In *Globalization, Neo-Conservative Policies and Democratic Alternatives: Essays in Honour of John Loxley*, edited by A. Sepheri, R. Chenomas, and A. H. Akra, 177–200. Winnipeg: Arbeiter Ring.

Serres, Michel. 2007. *The Parasite*. Minneapolis: University of Minnesota Press.

Shah, Sonia. 2016. "What You Get When You Mix Chickens, China and Climate Change." *New York Times*, February 5. http://www.nytimes.com/2016/02/07/opinion/sunday/what-you -get-when-you-mix-chickens-china-and-climate-change.html. Accessed October 3, 2017.

Sharp, Lesley A., and Nancy N. Chen, eds. 2014. *Bioinsecurity and Vulnerability*. Santa Fe, NM: School for Advanced Research Press.

Shohet, Merav. 2013. "Everyday Sacrifice and Language Socialization in Vietnam: The Power of a Respect Particle." *American Anthropologist* 115 (2): 203–17. https://doi.org/10.1111/aman .12004.

Shortridge, K. F., and C. H. Stuart-Harris. 1982. "An Influenza Epicentre?" *Lancet (London, England)* 2 (8302): 812–13.

Shukin, Nicole. 2009. *Animal Capital: Rendering Life in Biopolitical Times*. Minneapolis: University of Minnesota Press.

Sims, Les, and Huu Dung Do. 2009. "Vaccination of Poultry in Vietnam against H5N1 Highly Pathogenic Avian Influenza." Commonwealth of Australia. http://www.aitoolkit.org/site/ DefaultSite/filesystem/documents/CASE%20STUDY_07-09-09%20final.pdf. Accessed September 10, 2014.

Small, Ivan V. 2012. "'Over There': Imaginative Displacements in Vietnamese Remittance Gift Economies." *Journal of Vietnamese Studies* 7 (3): 157–83. https://doi.org/10.1525/vs.2012.7 .3.157.

Smallman, Shawn. 2013. "Biopiracy and Vaccines: Indonesia and the World Health Organization's New Pandemic Influenza Plan." *Journal of International and Global Studies* 4 (2): 20–36.

Smith, James, Emma Michelle Taylor, and Pete Kingsley. 2015. "One World-One Health and Neglected Zoonotic Disease: Elimination, Emergence and Emergency in Uganda." *Social Science & Medicine*, One World, One Health? Social science engagements with the one medicine agenda, 129 (March): 12–19. https://doi.org/10.1016/j.socscimed.2014.06.044.

Smith, Page, and Charles Daniel. 2000. *The Chicken Book.* Athens: University of Georgia Press.

Smithson, Paul. 1993. "Health Financing and Sustainability in Vietnam." Sustainability in the Health Sector Project. London: Save the Children Fund, UK.

Sontag, Susan. 1990. *Illness as Metaphor: and, AIDS and Its Metaphors.* New York: Doubleday.

Speedy, Andrew. 2008. "Speech by Mr Andrew Speedy, FAO Representative in Viet Nam at the Meeting to Review the Strategy for Control and Prevention of Highly Pathogenic Avian Influenza in the Agriculture Sector." Hanoi, August 13. UN speech. http://www.un.org.vn/en/fao-speeches/614-speech-by-mr-andrew-speedy-fao-representative-in-viet-nam-at-the-meeting-to-review-the-strategy-for-control-and-prevention-of-highly-pathogenic-avian-influenza-in-the-agriculture-sector.html. Accessed October 23, 2013.

Squier, Susan. 2012. *Poultry Science, Chicken Culture: A Partial Alphabet.* Newark, NJ: Rutgers University Press.

Stephenson, Niamh. 2011. "Emerging Infectious Disease/Emerging Forms of Biological Sovereignty." *Science, Technology & Human Values* 36 (5): 616–37. https://doi.org/10.1177/016224 3910388023.

Strathern, Marilyn. 2000. *Audit Cultures: Anthropological Studies in Accountability, Ethics and the Academy.* New York: Routledge.

Sunder Rajan, Kaushik. 2005. "Subjects of Speculation: Emergent Life Sciences and Market Logics in the United States and India." *American Anthropologist* 107 (1): 19–30.

———. 2006. *Biocapital: The Constitution of Postgenomic Life.* Durham, NC: Duke University Press.

———. 2017. *Pharmocracy: Value, Politics, and Knowledge in Global Biomedicine.* Durham, NC: Duke University Press.

Supari, Siti Fadilah. 2008. *It's Time for the World to Change: In the Spirit of Dignity, Equity, and Transparency; Divine Hand Behind Avian Influenza.* Jakarta: Sulaksana Watinsa.

Swayne, D. E., and E. Spackman. 2013. "Current Status and Future Needs in Diagnostics and Vaccines for High Pathogenicity Avian Influenza." *Developments in Biologicals* 135: 79–94. https://doi.org/10.1159/000325276.

Tai, Hue-Tam Ho. 1992. *Radicalism and the Origins of the Vietnamese Revolution.* Cambridge, MA: Harvard University Press.

———. 2001. *The Country of Memory: Remaking the Past in Late Socialist Vietnam.* Berkeley: University of California Press.

Tai, Hue-Tam Ho, and Mark Sidel. 2012. *State, Society and the Market in Contemporary Vietnam: Property, Power and Values.* London: Routledge.

Tanweer, Anissa, Brittany Fiore-Gartland, and Cecilia Aragon. 2016. "Impediment to Insight to Innovation: Understanding Data Assemblages through the Breakdown–Repair Process." *Information, Communication & Society* 19 (March): 1–17. https://doi.org/10.1080/1369118X .2016.1153125.

Taylor, Keith Weller. 1983. *The Birth of Vietnam.* Berkeley: University of California Press.

Taylor, Nora A. 2004. *Painters in Hanoi: An Ethnography of Vietnamese Art.* Honolulu: University of Hawai'i Press.

Taylor, Philip. 2000. *Fragments of the Present: Searching for Modernity in Vietnam's South.* Honolulu: University of Hawai'i Press.

———. 2007. "Poor Policies, Wealthy Peasants: Alternative Trajectories of Rural Development in Vietnam." *Journal of Vietnamese Studies* 2 (2): 3–56.

Thayer, Carlyle. 1992. "Political Reform in Vietnam: Doi Moi and the Emergence of Civil Society." In *The Developments of Civil Society in Communist Systems*, edited by Robert F. Miller. Sydney: Allen and Unwin.

Tran, Huu Bich, Van Truong Bui, and Ngoc Quang La. 2006. "A Meta-Evaluation of Avian Influenza Information, Education and Communication Studies and Knowledge, Attitude and Practice Surveys and Assessments in Vietnam 2003-2006." Hanoi: Hanoi School of Public Health.

Tsing, Anna Lowenhaupt. 2005. *Friction: An Ethnography of Global Connection.* Princeton, NJ: Princeton University Press.

———. 2012. "Unruly Edges: Mushrooms as Companion Species." *Environmental Humanities* 1: 141–54.

———. 2015. *The Mushroom at the End of the World: On the Possibility of Life in Capitalist Ruins.* Princeton, NJ: Princeton University Press.

Turner, Karen Gottschang. 1999. *Even the Women Must Fight: Memories of War from North Vietnam.* New York: Wiley.

United Nations. 1992. *United Nations Convention on Biological Diversity.* https://www.cbd.int/convention/text. Accessed July 13, 2013.

Vallat, Bernard. 2005. "Transparency on Avian Influenza Virus Strains: The OIE/FAO OFFLU Network; OIE—World Organisation for Animal Health." World Organization for Animal Health. 2005. http://www.oie.int/en/for-the-media/editorials/detail/article/transparency-on-avian-influenza-virus-strains-the-oiefao-offlu-network/. Accessed July 28, 2018.

Vezzani, Simone. 2010. "Preliminary Remarks on the Envisaged World Health Organization Pandemic Influenza Preparedness Framework for the Sharing of Viruses and Access to Vaccines and Other Benefits." *Journal of World Intellectual Property* 13 (6): 675–96. https://doi.org/10.1111/j.1747-1796.2010.00400.x.

Vivieros de Castro, Eduardo. 2004. "Perspectival Anthropology and the Method of Controlled Equivocation." *Tipití: Journal for the Society of Lowland South America* 2 (1): 3–22.

Vo, Ba. 2004. "Theo Chân Đội 'Săn Bắt Gà.'" *Thanh Nien: Diễn Đàn của Hội Liên Hiệp Thanh Niên Việt Nam*, February 9, sec. Chính Trị- Xã Hội. http://www.thanhnien.com.vn/news/Pages/200407/101201.aspx. Accessed Februrary 3, 2015.

Vu, Tuong. 2009. "The Political Economy of Avian Influenza Response and Control InVietnam." STEPS Working Paper 19. Brighton: STEPS Centre.

Waisbord, Silvio. 2001. "Communication for Social Change Consortium (CFSC Consortium)." May 30, 2001. http://www.communicationforsocialchange.org/publications-resources?itemid=21. Accessed June 6, 2014.

Wald, Priscilla. 2008. *Contagious: Cultures, Carriers, and the Outbreak Narrative.* 1st ed. Durham, NC: Duke University Press.

Waldby, Catherine, and Robert Mitchell. 2006. *Tissue Economies: Blood, Organs, and Cell Lines in Late Capitalism.* Durham, NC: Duke University Press.

Weaver, Harlan. 2013. "'Becoming in Kind': Race, Class, Gender, and Nation in Cultures of Dog Rescue and Dogfighting." *American Quarterly* 65 (3): 689–709. https://doi.org/10.1353/aq.2013.0034.

Wibisono, Makarim. 2008. "The Responsible Virus and Sharing Benefits." *Jakarta Post*, August 27, sec. Opinion. http://www.thejakartapost.com/news/2008/08/27/the-responsible-virus-and-sharing-benefits.html. Accessed May 29, 2014.

Willerslev, Rane. 2004. "Not Animal, Not Not-Animal: Hunting, Imitation and Empathic Knowledge among the Siberian Yukaghirs." *Journal of the Royal Anthropological Institute* 10 (3): 629–52.

Wolf, Meike, and Kevin Hall. 2018. "Cyborg Preparedness: Incorporating Knowing and Caring Bodies into Emergency Infrastructures." *Medical Anthropology* Advance Online Publication. https://doi.org/10.1080/01459740.2018.1485022.

Wolf-Meyer, Matthew J. 2017. "Normal, Regular, and Standard: Scaling the Body through Fecal Microbial Transplants." *Medical Anthropology Quarterly* 31 (3): 297–314. https://doi.org/10 .1111/maq.12328.

World Bank. 2018. "The World Bank in Vietnam." Text/HTML. http://www.worldbank.org/en/ country/vietnam/overview.

World Health Organization. 2011. "WHO: Pandemic Influenza Preparedness Framework for the Sharing of Influenza Viruses and Access to Vaccines and Other Benefits." World Health Organization. http://www.who.int/influenza/resources/pip_framework/en/.

———. 2016. "WHO: Cumulative Number of Confirmed Human Cases of Avian Influenza A(H5N1) Reported to WHO." http://www.who.int/influenza/human_animal_interface/ H5N1_cumulative_table_archives/en/. Accessed March 24, 2018.

World Organization for Animal Health. 2011. "Avian Influenza H5N1 Clade 2.3.2.1." World Organization for Animal Health: Press Releases. August 31. http://www.oie.int/for-the-media/ press-releases/detail/article/avian-influenza-h5n1-clade-2321/. Accessed December 22, 2015.

———. 2015. "Terrestrial Code: OIE—World Organisation for Animal Health." http://www.oie .int/en/international-standard-setting/terrestrial-code/. Accessed May 3, 2015.

Zhan, Mei. 2005. "Civet Cats, Fried Grasshoppers, and David Beckham's Pajamas: Unruly Bodies after SARS." *American Anthropologist* 107 (1): 31–42.

Index

social mobilization, 134; behavior change communications (BCC), 132; disease control, 121; global health programming, 132; political ends of, 121; of women, and sacrifice, 122
South Korea, 1. *See also* Korea
South Vietnam, 31, 122–23. *See also* North Vietnam; Vietnam
Soviet Union, 121, 198n4
Spackman, E., 165
Spanish Flu, 154, 199n1
spatial marginalization, 106
Speedy, Andrew, 73
Squier, Susan, 101
Standard Material Transfer Agreements (SMTAs), 153, 157. *See also* Material Transfer Agreements (MTAs)
Sunder Rajan, Kaushik, 155, 195n4
Supari, Siti Fadilah, 152, 154, 157, 166, 200n8
Swayne, D. E., 165
swine flu, 23

Taiwan, 33, 96
Taylor, Keith, 28–29
Taylor, Nora, 122
Taylor, Philip, 95
tethering, 153–55, 163, 166; moral ground, 164
Tết Lunar New Year: as dangerous holiday, 91–92; flu season, 91–92
Thailand, 2, 89–90, 101, 105, 155, 166
therapeutic clientship, 52
Thi Sách, 198n6
Three Priority Behaviors Campaign, 134–35, 138, 142, 145–46; behavior change intervention, 183
To Xuan Phuc, 197n10
Turner, Karen, 198n5

Uganda, 193–94n6
UNICEF, 116, 121; Avian Influenza Communications, 128, 197–98n1
United Kingdom, 36, 199n1. *See also* Britain
United Nations (UN), 12, 120, 168; Convention on Biological Diversity (CBD), 153–54, 199n2; Food and Agricultural Organization (FAO), 10, 15, 35, 37–38, 40, 42, 73, 89, 91–92, 105, 150–51, 157–61, 163, 165, 169, 200n8; Pro-Poor Livestock Policy Initiative, 94
United States, 36, 94, 138, 199n1, 200n10; social marketing, 133
urbanization, 32, 34
USAID, 11, 161

vaccination, 68–72, 74, 84, 105, 166, 182–83, 196n6; H5N1, 165; highly pathogenic avian influenza (HPAI), 63, 79, 83; life forms and forms of life, separation from, 65; of mass poultry, 25, 64–65, 177; Newcastle disease, 76, 78, 80–81,

200n11; and pandemics, 63, 76, 81–82. *See also* poultry vaccinations
Vertical Ray of the Sun, The (film), 112–13
Việt Minh (League of Independence of Vietnam), 198n2
Vietnam, 16, 18, 20, 23–24, 26, 40, 48, 50–51, 54–55, 63, 74–75, 82–84, 103–4, 116–17, 119, 135, 137–40, 142, 160, 162, 164–65, 175–78, 180, 183–85, 187–88; agricultural economy, shrinking of, 9; agricultural production, gains in, 8; avian flu aid, 10; avian flu strategy, 15, 65–66, 73; backyard chickens, 47, 56; *bao cấp* (subsidy system), 31–32; behavior change communications (BCC), 118; bird flu in, 13; bird flu control, 21; bird flu outbreaks, 2, 4, 11, 17; bird flu programmers, 37–38; capacity building, 166–67; chicken, symbolic role in, 28–29, 109, 111–13; chicken imagery in, 112, 114; chicken production, as scavenging farming systems, 46; chickens, formation of, 28; city and country, separation of in, 95–96, 106; commercializing economy, 95; democratic capitalism, 133–34; Department of Health (DAH), 158–59, 161; disease control, 94–95; *đổi mới* economic reforms, 8, 11–12, 32, 125; dual cosmos of thinking, 197n7; ethical variability, 201n1; famine in, 29; folk art (Đông Hồ woodblock printing), 122, 124; food insecurity, 29; foreign market investments, open to, 167; H5N1 virus outbreaks, 10, 12, 14, 25, 196n2; health care, 193n5; hyperinflation, 8; *hy sinh* (sacrifice), 109, 111; industrialization, 34, 87–89; industrialization and prosperity, tied to, 125, 128; infection, and surveillance systems, 195n1; Japanese invasion of, 29; kin-based poultry production, 99; livestock, idealized images of, 128; livestock economies, 173, 179; malaria control in, 195n3; market-based socialism, transition to, 118; market economy, changes in, 8; market restrictions, 86–90, 96, 105–7; and modernization, 128; National Institute of Hygiene and Epidemiology, 167; origins of, 28; "para-statal" partnerships, 179; place-based biological exchanges, as common, 97; poultry, cultural importance in, 109; poultry keeping, reliance on, 179; poultry markets, 85–86; poultry production, 4–5, 8–10; poultry restructuring in, 98; poultry vaccinations, 68–71; poultry value chains, 99; propaganda in, 122–23, 126, 128, 132; public health crisis in, 64; public health system, shifts in, 11; reunification of, 7–8, 31; revolutionary struggle, female involvement in, 198n6; rural economy, 32; sacrificial mother, theme of, 123; science, and health problems, 127–28; self-regulation, 146; self-responsibility, as social endeavor, 147; social mobilization, and